INFLAMMATORY BOWEL DISEASE
A Guide for Patients and Their Families

Inflammatory Bowel Disease
A Guide for Patients and Their Families

Stephen B. Hanauer, M.D.

Assistant Professor of Medicine
The Pritzker School of Medicine
The University of Chicago
Hospitals and Clinics
Chicago, Illinois

Joseph B. Kirsner, M.D., Ph.D.

Louis Block Distinguished Service
Professor of Medicine
The Division of the Biological Sciences
The Pritzker School of Medicine
The University of Chicago
Hospitals and Clinics
Chicago, Illinois

With Contributions By

Barbara S. Kirschner, M.D.

Associate Professor of Pediatrics
The Pritzker School of Medicine
The University of Chicago
Hospitals and Clinics
Chicago, Illinois

Janice C. Colwell, B.S.N., R.N.

Enterostomal Therapist
The University of Chicago
Hospitals and Clinics
Chicago, Illinois

Raven Press ■ New York

Raven Press, 1140 Avenue of the Americas, New York, New York 10036

© 1985 by Raven Press Books, Ltd. All rights reserved. This books is protected by copyright. No part of it may be reproduced, stored in a retrieval system, or transmitted, in any form or by any means, electronic, mechanical, photocopying, recording, or otherwise, without the prior written permission of the publisher.

Made in the United States of America

Library of Congress Cataloging in Publication Data

Hanauer, Stephen B.
   Inflammatory bowel disease.

   Includes bibliographies and index.
   1. Ulcerative colitis.   2. Enteritis, Regional.
I. Kirsner, Joseph B., 1909-   . II. Title.
[DNLM: 1. Colitis, Ulcerative.   2. Crohn Disease.
WI 522 H2333i]
RC862.C63H36   1985   616.3'44   84-24958
ISBN 0-89004-950-5
ISBN 0-88167-072-3 (soft)

To Our Families and Patients
It Is They Who Are Dedicated

Preface

All at present known in medicine is almost nothing in comparison with what remains to be discovered.
                                        René Descartes (1596–1650)

The "nonspecific" inflammatory bowel diseases, ulcerative colitis and Crohn's disease, until quite recently, were virtually unknown entities. Although ulcerative colitis had been described as early as 1859 in England, many of the early cases probably included forms of colitis. It was not until 1932, through the work of Drs. Crohn, Ginzburg, and Oppenheimer, that ilietis was defined as a separate entity. It is now apparent that the prevalence of these previously rare ailments has increased dramatically over the past several decades, such that thousands of Americans and hundreds of thousands of patients worldwide are affected.

There have been many advances in the scientific understanding of inflammatory bowel disease over the past 50 years, although no definitive cause or cure has been identified. Physicians, for example, are now capable of distinguishing certain bacteria, parasites, and viruses that may mimic inflammatory bowel disease, but that may be treated as an isolated incident. Researchers are hopeful that they, in the near future, will be able to produce or induce either Crohn's disease or ulcerative colitis in experimental situations, a major step toward finding a cure.

Inflammatory bowel disease (IBD) was once thought to be of emotional or psychosomatic origin. It is now obvious to the medical community that while stress certainly can aggravate the symptoms of IBD, no specific psychological factors initiate the disease process. Certainly, it is recognized that the illnesses themselves can produce emotional strains on the patients and their families, as is true for many chronic conditions.

After many years of treating IBD patients, we have evolved a truly comprehensive approach to the treatment of IBD. Rather than a trendy therapy involving "natural foods" and "homeopathic medicines," we emphasize the involvement of patients in their own care with family support, and advocate using the advances in medical knowledge to develop a program of treatment for each individual that incorporates nutrition and diet, recommendations for physical activity, lifestyle, and emotional support, in addition to standard medical (and, if necessary, surgical) treatment. All of these elements serve the long-term benefit of the "whole" individual.

This book is intended to provide introductory and basic information to allow patients and their families to better understand the scope of these illnesses, as well as to learn more about the specific aspects pertaining to individual problems. We introduce the basic terminology of IBD as well as provide a very general understanding of the anatomy and function of the gastrointestinal tract. We also discuss the causes of diarrheal illnesses that can mimic or complicate IBD. The various therapies are covered, including the types of medicine and treatment currently available for both Crohn's disease and ulcerative colitis. At all times, we emphasize the need for teamwork, and anticipate that this book will help patients and their families work hand-in-hand with their physician and the wider network of medical, surgical, nursing, dietary, pharmacy, social work, psychiatric, and religious professionals to be called on where and when necessary.

It is hoped that after reading this patient guide, you will be better able to comprehend the options available or recommendations offered by your medical "team" and be able to participate more fully in the decisions and care for yourself or for your loved-one.

Stephen B. Hanauer
Joseph B. Kirsner

Contents

INFLAMMATORY BOWEL DISEASE
A Guide for Patients and Their Families

CHAPTER 1

Introduction

The term inflammatory bowel disease refers to a group of illnesses affecting the gastrointestinal tract. Although the primary process,
inflammation, is usually confined to the digestive organs, the disease may affect almost any area of the body as an indirect consequence of the inflammation, or of the associated malnutrition and
infection, or as a result of the side effects of drugs prescribed for
treatment. An understanding of the varied manifestations of inflammatory bowel disease requires knowledge of the normal digestive
tract, its anatomy, its functions, and how the particular problems
interfere with its normal activities. Some definitions are required
initially to enable you to comprehend fully the material that follows.

The gastrointestinal (GI) tract refers to the continuous tube that
extends from the mouth to the anus (Fig. 1).[1] The inner layer of the
digestive tube is actually outside of the body, since both ends are
open to the environment. The basic function of the digestive tract is
to allow nutrients necessary for normal functioning and survival to
enter the body while excluding and eliminating unnecessary or
harmful substances. The GI tract extends from the head (at the
mouth) through the neck and chest (via the *esophagus*) into the
abdomen. The abdominal segments include the *stomach, small in-*

---

[1]This refers to the tubular portion of the digestive tract. The liver, gallbladder,
and pancreas also are constituents of the digestive tract but are not the principal
targets of inflammatory bowel disease.

1

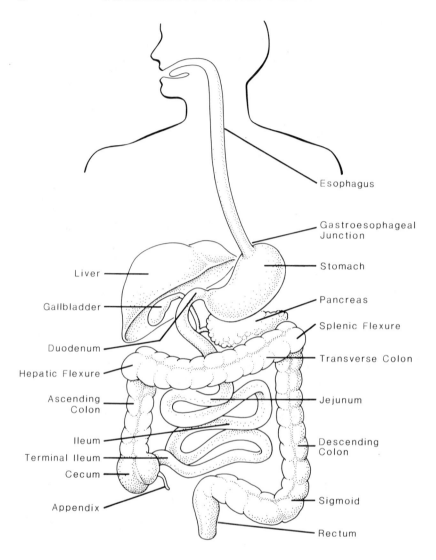

FIG. 1. Anatomy of the gastrointestinal tract.

testine, and *large intestine* (colon). The last portion of the colon is the *rectum*, which ends at the *anal sphincter* (anus).

The GI tract is actually a group of hollow organs arranged in several layers (see Fig. 2). The *lumen* refers to the inner space within the bowel containing the intestinal contents. The innermost

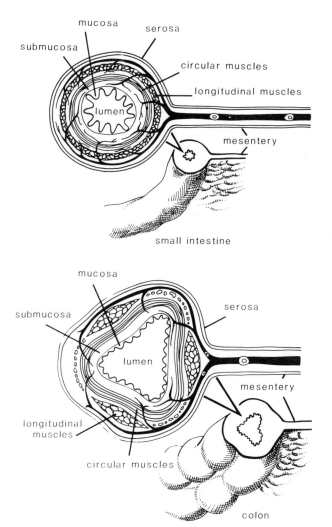

FIG. 2. The layers of the GI tract that make up the bowel wall. **Top:** Small intestine; **bottom:** colon.

layer is the *mucosa*, which is lined by special cells characteristic of the individual segment of the tract (stomach, small intestine, or colon) that function to produce enzymes for the digestion of food and absorption of appropriate luminal contents; other cells produce *mucus* to lubricate and protect the inner surface from harmful material. Supporting the mucosa is the *submucosa*, a layer of several cell types, nerves, and blood vessels. The submucosa further samples the absorbed material and transports nutrients into the body or defends against foreign or potentially harmful material that may have crossed through the mucosal barrier. The next layers are two sets of *smooth muscle* (a special type of muscle with its own rhythmic contractions). The muscle closest to the inner surface is a circular band; the outer core is composed of longitudinal strands. The muscular layers contract in sequence to churn and mix the bowel contents or to propel them down the tube. The propulsive movement in the gut is termed *peristalsis*. External to the muscle is the *serosal* layer of supporting tissue, which connects the various segments of the digestive tube to other organs, to blood vessels, or to the lining inside of the abdominal wall, the *peritoneal cavity*.

Inflammation applies to the reaction against infecting or damaging agents. The inflammatory process is characterized by vascular congestion and swelling of the tissues, and involves special white blood cells that defend the body against foreign compounds (called antigens). The inflammatory cells include several types of white blood cells—polymorphonuclear leukocytes, lymphocytes, and plasma cells—as well as special types of cells in the tissue such as macrophages and mast cells. These cells are part of the immune system and function to recognize normal body components and to react against elements foreign or harmful to the body. To do so, they produce chemicals that can damage the surrounding tissue and also attract more inflammatory cells to the location of the tissue injury. In this manner, the local response is often amplified in order to defend against the action of potentially dangerous material such as abnormal bacteria. These cells may also inadvertently damage the local structures of the gut if the reaction goes ''out of control'' or becomes self-perpetuating.

Although the different cell types involved in the inflammatory response are usually able to halt further injury when the foreign material has been neutralized, at times the inflammation may result in more damage than would have been produced by the foreign substances. In special circumstances, these cells react against normal body tissue components as if they were foreign in a process called an *autoimmune reaction*. Immunologically mediated processes are being intensely investigated as potential causes of inflammatory bowel disease and similar autoimmune disorders.

Any inflammatory reaction within the intestinal tract has several possible consequences. The basic response is *edema* or swelling caused by the leakage of fluid from the damaged blood vessels into the tissues. *Ulcerations* (disruptions of the surface lining) of varying size develop if the intestine is so injured that the lining cells are damaged or destroyed, creating a break in the mucosal barrier. The supporting cells and vessels are then exposed to the luminal contents and will often leak tissue fluid and blood. When ulcers penetrate deeply into the more external layers of the intestine they are called *fissures*, in essence, deeper knife-like cracks. In some instances, the inflammation can involve the entire thickness of the bowel wall. If this occurs, another loop of bowel usually will move alongside the inflamed segment. The inflammatory reactions may burrow into an adjacent segment of bowel, creating a *fistula* or abnormal connection, usually at a point of ulceration or fissure. Fistulas can also develop between bowel and skin or between bowel and any other abdominal structure, including the urinary system (bladder or ureter) and the genital tract (ovaries, uterus, vagina).

When inflammation subsides in the gut, the healing response usually involves some scarring from the deposits of fibrous tissue in damaged areas. The scar tissue is not as elastic or flexible as normal tissue and may cause a partial narrowing of the gut if the healing process leaves the wall of the intestine thickened to the point of impinging on the lumen. This narrowing is called a *stricture*, and, depending on the diameter of the lumen, can impede the normal transit of intestinal contents, or even produce total obstruction. Similar fibrous bands within the abdomen are termed *adhesions* and usually develop after abdominal operations; these form attachments between different portions of the intestinal wall, resulting in a kinking of loops of the bowel or interference with the usual fluid movement of the intestines.

DEFINITIONS

Inflammatory bowel disease is a general term applicable to several different disease processes manifested as inflammation of the bowel. The inflammatory reaction may be attributable to a known cause, e.g., infectious agents (viruses, bacteria, parasites), toxins to a particular area of the bowel, autoimmune reactions, radiation damage, or, especially in older people, defective blood supply. When none of these conditions are present or identified, there remains a group of diseases that are considered *idiopathic* (the cause is not known). The latter can be further grouped descriptively by the segment of bowel involved, the associated symptoms, complications, natural history, and/or response to the treatment. The idiopathic inflammatory bowel diseases consist of ulcerative colitis and Crohn's disease. Both illnesses are considered *chronic* (conditions that tend to persist or to recur despite treatment), and since treatment is not specific, they are regarded as controllable rather than curable disorders.

Ulcerative Colitis

Ulcerative colitis is an inflammation of the *colon* (large intestine or bowel). The inflammation is confined to the colon in all instances and never spreads to other areas of the intestines. The inflammatory reaction usually involves only the more superficial layer of the intestine (the mucosa), and deep, penetrating ulcers or fistulas do not occur. The superficial inflammation usually begins in the rectum which is involved in almost all cases. When the inflammation spreads to other portions of the colon, it does so in a diffusely continuous fashion without skipping segments. Hence, once the inflammation has spread from the rectum, the areas downstream remain affected in continuity with the rectum. Conversely, healing occurs first from the segments further from the rectum and also proceeds as a continuous process.

The earliest microscopic changes are dilations (widening) of blood vessels and increased blood supply to the lining of the colon. Later, pinpoint ulcerations occur in the lining of the colon with a propensity to bleeding such that gentle wiping of the wall with a

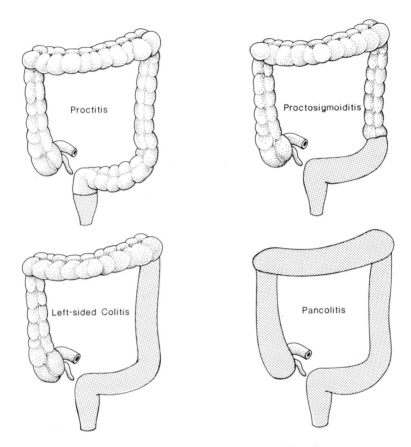

FIG. 3. The forms of ulcerative colitis. Areas affected by disease are represented by shading.

cotton swab produces blood. Later, as the process advances, the ulcerations can become more prominent and confluent. These always remain superficial and almost never penetrate through the intestinal wall except in very severe, rapidly progressive (fulminating) disease.

When the inflammatory process is confined to the rectum, the condition is known as *proctitis* or ulcerative proctitis. If the inflammation does not extend beyond the descending colon, it is called left-sided colitis. When the entire colon is involved, the condition is termed *pancolitis* (see Fig. 3). The extent of the disorders does not necessarily reflect the degree of activity of the inflammation. For instance, a patient with proctitis may have severe symptoms and bleeding, whereas another individual with the entire colon involved (pancolitis) may be in a state of healing and present few or no symptoms.

Crohn's Disease

Whereas ulcerative colitis is a continuous and relatively superficial form of inflammation of the bowel's inner surface, Crohn's disease refers to an inflammatory process that is characteristically focal (involving discrete areas separated by normal portions of the

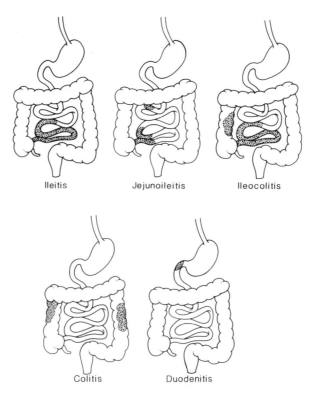

Ileitis	Jejunoileitis	Ileocolitis

Colitis	Duodenitis

FIG. 4. Patterns of Crohn's disease. Areas affected by disease are represented by shading.

GI tract), affects the deeper layers of the bowel wall, and is capable of producing fissures and fistulas. Whereas ulcerative colitis is limited to the colon, Crohn's disease can involve any portion of the gastrointestinal tract from the mouth to the anus. Various synonyms for Crohn's disease relate to the portion of the bowel that is affected and to the special type of inflammation that may produce granulomas (collections of special inflammatory cells). *Terminal ileitis* refers to Crohn's disease limited to the last portion of the small bowel (ileum). *Regional enteritis* implies that the Crohn's disease involves several areas within the small intestine. *Granulomatous colitis* refers to Crohn's disease involving the colon. Other common descriptive terms include *jejunoileitis*, which means that both the jejunum (first half of the small intestine) and ileum are involved, or *ileocolitis* if both the ileum and colon have changes caused by Crohn's disease (Fig. 4).

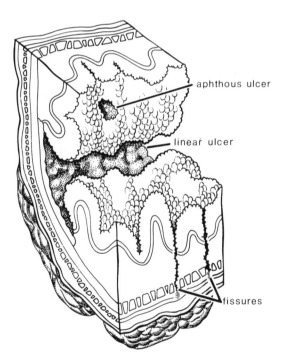

FIG. 5. Mucosal lesions of Crohn's disease.

The initial microscopic changes of Crohn's disease involve pinpoint ulcerations called aphthoid ulcers located on top of lymphoid follicles (groupings of lymphocytes) distributed throughout the GI tract (Fig. 5). These ulcers enlarge and frequently deepen to produce linear ulcers or fissures, which can burrow through the layers of the intestinal wall. Fistulas occur when the inflammation traverses through the bowel wall into an adjacent loop of intestine. Unlike ulcerative colitis, a segment of severely inflamed bowel can be found immediately adjacent to a completely normal segment; hence, the focal nature of Crohn's disease. Microscopic changes of Crohn's disease often are found in segments of bowel far removed from any disease activity. Even though active Crohn's disease may be confined to focal segments of the gut, the inflammatory process may involve the entire gastrointestinal tract, although subtly so no obvious symptoms or gross changes are produced.

CHAPTER 2

The Cause of Inflammatory Bowel Disease

INFECTIONS

The cause, or etiology, of inflammatory bowel disease has not yet been determined. Ever since these illnesses were first described, investigators have searched for infectious agents, either bacteria or viruses. Although numerous bacteria (see Chapter 3) can produce identical symptoms and pathologic changes to those found in ulcerative colitis or Crohn's disease, major differences include the self-limited course of the bacterial infections as well as the immediate response to antibiotic treatment. Furthermore, in infectious colitis, the lining (mucosa) of the colon returns completely to normal after treatment, whereas with ulcerative colitis, even during a complete remission of symptoms, microscopic changes continue to be observed.

Investigators have searched for bacterial and viral agents by culturing the contents of the stool of patients with ulcerative colitis, by microscopic examination of the gut wall looking for invasion by bacteria, by electron microscopic examination of individual cells lining the intestinal tract, and by testing for serum and intestinal antibody responses to individual bacteria and viruses. The magnitude of the problem can be understood a bit better if you consider that there are over 10 billion bacteria per gram of fecal contents. There are over 100 different strains of bacteria, each with its own growth characteristics and requirements, making identification and

11

enumeration of each species of bacteria in any one individual's intestinal contents a monumental task. To do so for a group of patients is logistically impossible. Hence, it is routine practice to culture the intestinal contents only for known potential bacterial or viral causes of inflammation when an individual has ileitis or colitis.

Physicians are constantly identifying new types of bacteria and viral infections of the intestinal tract. Subtle differences in the presentation and course of various illnesses give clues to investigators that they may be dealing with a new infectious agent. In this way, *Campylobacter*, a recently recognized bacterial strain, has been identified as a frequent cause of infectious colitis. Descriptive information regarding the nature of human infections caused by this organism has been available only for the past 10 years. Likewise, infections caused by *Yersinia enterocolitica* may completely mimic Crohn's ileitis aside from the discriminating feature of complete resolution of the *Yersinia* ileitis. Crohn's disease does not heal by itself or with antibiotics alone. Physicians also only recently have become aware that rectal disease in homosexuals can be transmitted by various bacteria [*Campylobacter, Shigella, Gonorrhea, Chlamydia, Treponema pallidum* (syphilis)], parasites (*Amoeba, Giardia*), and viruses (herpes, cytomegalovirus). All of these have been explored as possible causative agents in inflammatory bowel disease; however, none has been consistently identified in patients.

Most recently, investigators have been on the trail of a variant strain of a bacterium similar to tuberculosis. An "atypical" mycobacterium has been cultured from a patient with Crohn's disease and transmitted to goats. Whether this bug will turn out to be a causative agent, or not, will require much further investigation involving a great many more patients and laboratory experiments.

Other possible sources of inflammation in these illnesses are toxins derived from bacteria or the environment. Some bacteria produce toxins that cause colitis. *Clostridium difficile* has been identified as the causative agent in many episodes of diarrhea that develop after the administration of antibiotics. This is because of suppression by antibiotics of normal gut bacteria that, under unusual circumstances, inhibit the growth of the *Clostridium difficile* organism. When antibiotics eliminate the normal bacteria, *Clostrid-*

ium difficile grows and produces the toxin. There are many other potential bacterial toxins that have yet to be identified; however, to date, research methods to identify toxins have not discovered a specific toxin in individuals afflicted with ulcerative colitis or Crohn's disease. The study of bacterial toxins continues to be a fertile area of investigation and needs to be expanded to include nonbacterial toxins.

DIETARY FACTORS

Certain food products (e.g., carageenan) have been shown to cause colitis in laboratory animals. Unfortunately, the illness produced in guinea pigs does not replicate either ulcerative colitis or Crohn's disease in humans. The absence of a true animal model of inflammatory bowel disease is a major handicap in investigating the disease and its treatment. If we had such an investigational tool, it would be possible to sample various infectious agents and toxins in laboratory animals and in this manner study further in the laboratory these unique conditions. To our knowledge, neither ulcerative colitis nor Crohn's disease affects any species other than humans.

You may have read about population studies that implicate various diets as predisposing to inflammatory bowel disease. These studies are very popular in the lay press and seem to get a great deal more attention than is warranted by the scientific basis (or lack thereof) of these investigations. Most of these studies have been done with small groups of patients and are poorly controlled for other confounding variables. For instance, one European group has implicated sugar as a factor in the development of Crohn's disease. The study seems to demonstrate that individuals with Crohn's disease eat more refined sugar than patients without the disease. The study fails to take into consideration the observation that individuals with Crohn's disease are often underweight because of their illness and that most products high in refined sugar are usually high in calories and easy to digest. Hence, it is reasonable for individuals with Crohn's disease to adapt their diet toward sugar-containing products as a "self-treatment," occurring not before but after the onset of the illness. Since so many people with Crohn's disease have an insidious onset, it is often difficult to document the beginning of such a diet before the first symptoms of inflammatory bowel disease. Particular foods such as corn flakes and margarine have been suggested as potential causes of inflammatory bowel disease, but there is no conclusive evidence. You should be aware that despite the popularity of such items in the nonscientific media, they frequently are misleading and without substantial scientific basis.

One such potentially dangerous implication involves fiber and inflammatory bowel disease. With the recent popularity of high-fiber diets in our society, some observers have suggested that patients with inflammatory bowel disease consume too little fiber in their diet. There is no evidence that high-fiber diets protect against inflammatory bowel disease, and there are many reasons why they should be avoided in patients with inflammatory bowel disease.

FAMILY AND GENETIC DATA

Both ulcerative colitis and Crohn's disease have been found to occur more frequently in families in which one member is known to be affected. This has led researchers to look for a genetic means of inheritance. To date, many studies have confirmed that inflammatory bowel disease does occur more frequently in some families. Between 20 and 40% of individuals who develop inflammatory bowel disease will have another family member with inflammatory bowel disease. Interestingly, there may be mixtures of Crohn's disease and ulcerative colitis in members of a single family. Offspring of an individual with inflammatory bowel disease also have an increased chance of developing ulcerative colitis or Crohn's disease, although there is no particular male or female preponderance, and there are, as yet, no means of identifying individual members at risk. Additionally, no evidence exists for direct transmission of inflammatory bowel disease within a family as might occur with an infection.

Attempts have been made to identify genetic markers associated with inflammatory bowel disease. You may have read about the HLA system in man, which is utilized in patients who receive organ transplants. The HLA system refers to a set of chemical markers occurring on human blood cells that are determined directly by a chromosome (gene) that regulates the immunologic response. Much work already had been completed attempting to compare various HLA types with the risk of developing inflammatory bowel diseases, but no such markers have been identified. Studies are under way that explore alternative genetic markers.

IMMUNOLOGY

The immunology of inflammatory bowel disease has been one of the most actively studied areas of these complex illnesses. Millions of dollars have been spent in attempting to define an immunologic cause for inflammatory bowel disease. Briefly, the immune response is the body's mechanism for recognizing what is part of one's self and what is foreign to the individual. The body must recognize foreign material and destroy or eliminate such substances while not damaging one of its own components. In this manner, bacteria and viruses are prevented from entering the internal environment of the body while necessary food particles can be absorbed. If the immune system is inadequate or disrupted, infectious agents or toxic substances can enter the body, or host, and cause damage. At the other extreme, if the host begins to react against its own components (an autoimmune reaction), normal tissue or structures can be injured.

Many disturbances of the immune system have been recognized in inflammatory bowel disease. However, no such disturbance has been found to occur prior to the development of the illness. In other words, there is no way to predict with immunologic tools which individual will eventually develop inflammatory bowel disease. It appears that most of the abnormalities that have been identified occur only after the individual has developed the inflammatory condition. Many are secondary to the underlying inflammation, and other immune abnormalities are related to secondary manifestations of inflammatory bowel disease such as malnutrition, treatment with medications, or surgery. Some disturbances may be related to the breakdown of the normal intestinal barrier that protects against invasion by gut bacterial populations.

Although no definitive immunological abnormality has yet been identified, this realm has exciting potential for identifying disease mechanisms as well as having therapeutic implications. Many of the medications used to treat inflammatory bowel disease directly or indirectly influence the immune system, and with a greater understanding of how this system operates in inflammatory bowel disease, we will eventually be able to fine tune a patient's immune response to react effectively against inflammation without jeopardizing its protective role.

CHAPTER 3

The Anatomy of the Gastrointestinal Tract

The gastrointestinal tract originates in the mouth. Here, digestion begins (discussed in Chapter 4) with the physical breakdown of large food portions into smaller particles by the teeth. At the same time, as food enters the mouth, secretions from the salivary gland begin chemically to break down smaller food particles into even smaller fragments preparatory to further processing in the intestines. When mixed and churned by the tongue and eventually swallowed, the soft masses of chewed food are now lubricated and pass into the esophagus. (You will find it helpful to refer to Fig. 1, page 2, showing the anatomy of the GI tract.)

The esophagus is a transport tube in the chest extruding from the pharynx to the stomach that directs the food from the oral cavity (mouth) into the stomach. Along its course the esophagus passes behind the lungs and the heart.

The junction of the esophagus and stomach (gastroesophageal junction) is at the diaphragm, separating the chest from the abdomen. The diaphragm is a large, flat muscle that moves rhythmically to expand the lungs and maintain respiration. Fibers of the diaphragmatic muscle surrounding the esophagus at the connection with the stomach provide a form of sphincter or valve control, which ordinarily prevents the backflow of food material from the stomach into the esophagus.

The stomach is a large reservoir in which the swallowed food collects and mixes further with the acid secretions. The acid content of the stomach eliminates most bacteria that may have been swallowed and continues the process of breaking down larger food particles into smaller and more basic components. The stomach also produces pepsin, an enzyme that begins to digest protein into smaller amino acid constituents. The stomach mixes the food until it is liquefied.

From the stomach, the liquid contents are slowly delivered via the exit point of the stomach (the pylorus) into the first portion of the small intestine, the *duodenum*. Here, the gastric contents are mixed with bile from the liver and enzyme secretions from the pancreas in addition to the secretions produced by the intestine. These chemicals continue the digestion process by reducing the large chains of carbohydrates, fats, and proteins to individual sugars, fatty acids, and amino acids, which can be absorbed more readily from the small intestine.

The small intestine continues from the duodenum as the *jejunum*. The jejunum is the main segment of the small intestine and absorbs into the bloodstream the majority of the simple nutrients that now lie within the intestinal lumen.

There is no distinct structural separation between the jejunal portion of the small intestine and the next segment, the *ileum*. The ileum not only continues the absorptive process of sugars, fatty acids, and amino acids that have escaped absorption in the jejunum, but it also contains a specialized area for the absorption of fat-soluble vitamins (vitamins A, D, E, and K), vitamin B_{12}, and bile salts.

The entire small intestine ranges from 12 to 20 feet in length. Because the lining surface is convoluted into tiny folds called villi, the entire absorptive surface is enormous. There also is an excess of small intestine so that individuals can easily survive even if 50% of the small bowel is diseased or surgically removed. If, however, the last portion of the ileum (terminal ileum) is absent, there may be inadequate absorption of the fat-soluble vitamins and vitamin B_{12}. The inadequate absorption of bile salts results in other problems (as described subsequently).

The terminal ileum empties into the first portion of the large intestine (colon), the *cecum*. Projecting from the top of the cecum lies the fingerlike projection of the appendix, in man a vestige of the lymphoid portion of the immune system; it has no known essential function. Material entering the colon at this point is in liquid form. The function of the colon is to absorb salt and water into the body. This process gradually allows a solidification of the bowel contents and, in the left colon, the completion of the stool formation. Material passes as a liquid through the ascending and transverse colon and only becomes more solid in the descending and sigmoid portions of the colon. The circular muscle layer of the colon is similar to that in the small intestine. However, the longitudinal muscle layer is separated into three distinct bands, or taenae. The taenae allow the colon to segment and further churn the intestinal contents as water is being absorbed until a peristaltic sequence of muscular action passes the fecal material into the rectum. When this material impacts on the rectum, nerve receptors are stimulated and initiate the urge to defecate. This is a conditioned response, involving relaxation of the anal sphincter and contraction of the abdominal muscles. This action enhances the muscular action of the rectum and anal sphincter to allow the purge of a compact, solid bowel movement.

CHAPTER 4

The Function of the
Gastrointestinal Tract

There are two primary functions of the gastrointestinal tract, the process of digestion and the maintenance of immunological mechanisms.

DIGESTION

The term digestion refers both to the breakdown of large food particles into component parts and to the absorption of the smaller basic food units. These basic units are categorized as proteins, carbohydrates, fats, minerals, and vitamins.

Proteins

Proteins are a basic building block of most plant and animal cells. They are present in greatest amounts in foods obtained from animals (meats and milk products) and certain vegetables. Proteins themselves are made up of basic units called *amino acids*. These are linked together in long chains, which twist around themselves to form three-dimensional structures that serve many life functions. In body tissues they form the foundation of muscle fibers and serve regulatory functions in controlling cellular activity and metabolic behavior.

The digestion of proteins begins in the mouth by the grinding action of teeth. In the stomach, the acid environment further divides the proteins into long chains of amino acids. An enzyme in the stomach called pepsin helps to separate these longer chains of amino acids into somewhat shorter chains. When the gastric contents are emptied into the duodenum (see Chapter 3), secretions from the pancreas including the enzymes trypsin and chymotrypsin break down the long chains of amino acids into single amino acids. These are then absorbed throughout the small intestine into the body, where they are utilized by the liver, muscle, or brain, and where they are reassimilated into larger protein structures that the body requires for its various functions.

Carbohydrates

Carbohydrates are long chains of *simple sugars*. The simple sugars most commonly ingested by man include glucose, sucrose (a combination of glucose and fructose), and milk sugar, lactose (a combination of glucose and galactose). Starches are long chains of glucose attached end to end in a special pattern. Cellulose, or plant fiber, is glucose united in another array.

Sugars, like amino acids, need to be broken down into single units to be absorbed from the intestine. In the mouth, the teeth break down larger units, which are then mixed with secretions from the salivary gland containing amylase, an enzyme that divides long chains of sugars when they are arranged as starches. Pancreatic secretions, also containing amylase further shorten these longer chains into either single sugars (monosaccharides) or double sugars (disaccharides). The cells lining the small intestine contain enzymes that cleave the disaccharides into single units, and the lining cells of the intestine then absorb these single sugars into the body.

Fats

Just as proteins and carbohydrates are composed of smaller units, fats consist of long chains of fatty acids that are united in groups of three, usually onto a simple backbone, as units called triglycerides. Because fats do not dissolve in water, bile salts are needed to render triglycerides more soluble in order for enzymes from the pancreas (lipases) to separate the fats into the fatty acids. The fatty acids are then absorbed from the small intestine. The bile salts also are re-absorbed from the ileum, circulate back to the liver, and are rese-creted into the bile (the so-called recycling process via the enterohepatic circulation).

Minerals and Vitamins

Minerals include all of the salts and other trace elements required to maintain the chemical equilibrium within the body fluids and individual cells. They also function as ingredients (or coenzymes) in assisting other proteins or enzymes to function appropriately. The great majority of these are absorbed in the jejunum.

Vitamins are more complex chemicals also required for the individual functioning of cells. The individual vitamins are described below (see Chapter 8). Vitamins are classified as those soluble in fat (vitamin A, D, E, and K) and those soluble in water (e.g., thiamine, pyridoxine, vitamin B_{12}, vitamin C, and niacin). The water-soluble vitamins, except for vitamin B_{12}, are absorbed in the jejunum. Vitamin B_{12} requires a protein (intrinsic factor) produced in the stomach to be absorbed from the terminal ileum. The fat-soluble vitamins also are absorbed from the terminal ileum.

Thus, abnormalities in any area of the gastrointestinal tract can influence the digestion and absorption of these essential nutrients. For instance, the absence of teeth or the inability to chew would affect the initial digestion of proteins and starches. Abnormalities in the stomach can alter the digestion of proteins, fats, and carbohydrates as well as vitamin B_{12}. Abnormalities of the pancreas may affect processing of all basic food groups. Those of the liver will influence the absorption of fat and fat-soluble vitamins. Intestinal dysfunction may modify the digestion and absorption of all basic food groups depending on the area of the intestine involved.

IMMUNOLOGY

A main function of the gastrointestinal tract is to sample from the environment those substances that are necessary to sustain life while excluding unnecessary, toxic, or harmful material. Just beneath and between the absorptive cells of the intestine lies an array of immune cells whose function it is to recognize substances foreign to the host and to prevent their entry into the body.

At birth lymphocytes, other immunologically active cells, and antibodies derived from the mother, are present in breast milk. This resource provides the initial protection of the infant from substances that may be harmful and to which the newborn has yet to be exposed. Later, with the more complete development of the various cells and membranes, the immunologically reactive cells recognize harmful substances that can be ingested by individual cells and renders them harmless by chemical processing. Other immune cells produce antibodies, which bind to the foreign substance (e.g., proteins, bacteria, viruses) and facilitate its metabolism in an innocuous fashion by scavenger cells (such as macrophages) within the wall of the intestine, liver, or spleen.

Breaches in this first immune barrier can occur when the mucosa of the intestine is injured. This may allow noxious material to be absorbed from the intestine and enter the circulatory system. A second filtering function is then performed by the *lymphatic* system, which is composed of small vessels that carry lymphocytes and drain into lymph nodes, which are small filters that consist of groupings (or follicles) of lymphocytes and other immune cells that together handle foreign proteins and particles as they circulate through the node. Examples of such useful structures are the tonsils in the throat or the lymph nodes we sometimes feel under the arms or in the neck. Additionally, any *antigens*, i.e., foreign compounds that are absorbed into the circulation are then filtered a third time through the liver, which is also well endowed with immune cells to deal with the foreign material.

Intestinal inflammation may influence the immune response by altering the intestinal barrier and allowing foreign or noxious substances to be absorbed more readily through defects in the intestinal wall. Malnutrition occurring in the setting of inflammatory bowel disease may also influence the body's immune response, which requires adequate protein and mineral stores to function properly.

Consequently, infections occur more often in undernourished individuals. Thus, the complicated interrelationships of the body's defense systems, ongoing inflammation, and complications of the inflammation can influence the outcome of any illness significantly.

In an individual already compromised by inflammatory bowel disease and complicated by maldigestion and malabsorption, an *adequate nutritional intake is essential* to restore body defenses to be able to deal with the increased exposure to noxious intestinal contents. At the same time, medical treatment is instituted to sustain the immune response and control the inflammatory process.

This extremely complex and usually well-functioning system is able to discriminate among millions of compounds that the intestine comes in contact with on a day-in and day-out basis. This system allows billions and billions of bacteria to exist within the intestine and yet prevents them from infiltrating into body tissue. Yet, all necessary food compounds, vitamins, minerals, and even medications can be absorbed without inducing a negative reaction. Medical scientists only now are learning the intricacies of the immune system's operation, which appears to hold great potential for further insight into the mode of development of inflammatory bowel disease. Furthermore, many of the medical therapies of inflammatory bowel disease directly or indirectly influence the immunologic response of the body. Medications such as corticosteroids reduce the inflammatory response. But at the same time, they can interfere with the defense mechanism protecting against foreign material. It is often this delicate balance that your physician is considering during the long-term treatment of inflammatory bowel disease.

CHAPTER 5

Diarrhea

Because diarrhea is such a prominent symptom of inflammatory bowel disease, it is worthwhile to discuss other causes of diarrhea that may be confused with inflammatory bowel disease or may complicate the course of the illness. In simplest terms, diarrhea is a change in bowel habits to looser or more frequent stools. Hence, someone who normally has a single formed bowel movement every 3 days and who begins to have a bowel movement daily may consider this diarrhea, whereas an individual with three mushy stools a day may consider this normal.

Actually, the number of bowel movements depends on diet, and norms differ between industrialized and less Westernized cultures. In the Western world, where consumption of meat and processed food makes up the "bulk" of the diet, there is less available roughage and fiber to hold fluid in stools, which then become more compact and less frequent. In African villages where vegetables and unprocessed foods are consumed more regularly, the bowel movements are larger, softer, and more frequent. The "normal" range of bowel movements in America and England is between 3 and 20 bowel movements per week. For instance, anywhere from one bowel movement every 3 days to 3 bowel movements a day probably is normal depending on the individual pattern.

Diarrhea also can be defined in medical terms. This depends more on the actual weight of the stool and the amount of water eliminated. The medical definition does not depend on the frequency or consistency of the stools. Diarrhea is defined in medical terms as the

27

production of more than 200 grams of stool water daily. This is the equivalent of approximately 6 to 8 oz of water daily.

There are many causes of diarrhea unrelated to inflammatory bowel disease. Most commonly, a temporary alteration in stool frequency can be attributed to changes in diet and may be related to the consumption of foods that are irritating to the bowel (highly seasoned or spicy foods, which stimulate the intestines to enhanced motility in order to eliminate the contents), foods that contain large amounts of undigestible products, such as roughage or fiber, which retain additional stool water, or meals containing large quantities of foods that are beyond the normal capacity of digestion at one time (such as large, fatty meals). Any of these will lead to an increased number of bowel movements.

Each individual has his or her own tolerance of foods. Some persons are more sensitive to all of the ingredients of food (including spices, fiber, and chemicals such as caffeine) and will always have a tendency to have more frequent bowel movements. At one extreme, we consider these individuals to have the "irritable bowel syndrome" in which the gastrointestinal system is more sensitive to all the stimuli that normally influence the gut (including foods, chemicals, body hormones, infections, and emotional or stress factors). In these individuals, many factors work singly or in combination to produce more frequent or uncomfortable bowel movements.

A common form of diarrhea in the general population is that caused by ingestion of milk products after the ability to digest the milk sugar lactose has been lost. Many populations lose the ability to break down the double sugar (disaccharide) lactose into the simple sugars glucose and galactose, which are then absorbed across the lining of the intestine. Lactose is then transported down the small intestine into the large bowel, where the normal bacteria ferment the sugars into gas and acid by-products, which are irritating to the colon and produce flatus and looser bowel movements. This problem can be easily managed by avoiding large amounts of milk products or by adding the enzyme lactase, which is now available as LactAid® or Lactase™, to milk before using it in foods or in baking. Acidophilus milk contains *Lactobacillus acidophilus*, which is capable of partially degrading lactose in the carton, and hence contains somewhat less lactose. However, this bacteria is only active in warm temperatures and is not very effective in breaking down lactose when cooled. Hence, when milk is refrigerated, the *Lactobacillus* does not convert very much lactose, and patients who are intolerant of the milk sugar will commonly continue to notice symptoms. Yogurt also is produced by using the same bacterium and contains somewhat less of the milk sugar lactose than regular milk.

INFECTIOUS DIARRHEA

Millions of individuals worldwide, mostly children, are affected by infectious diarrhea, which causes thousands of deaths yearly. Most of these occur in third world countries where sanitary conditions are substandard. Yet even in Westernized countries, diarrhea accounts for frequent episodes of illness and loss of time from work or school. Additionally, as worldwide travel has increased, diarrhea in travelers has become a most common occurrence. Recent outbreaks of diarrhea caused by *Salmonella* and by *Giardia* illustrate this point.

Infections can cause diarrhea by a variety of mechanisms. Some infectious agents interfere with the cells lining the intestine so that the simple nutrients cannot be absorbed. These nutrients will then pass into the colon, retaining water in the stool, or, are converted by the normal bacteria in the stool to products that are irritating and produce exaggerated motility or cause stimulation of fluid secretion into the bowel. Other infectious agents can invade the intestinal lining and establish an inflammatory response, which both impairs absorption of nutrients and, at the same time, causes the loss of blood and body fluids into the stool. Still other infectious agents produce toxins that stimulate secretion of fluid into the gut without evoking an inflammatory reaction.

VIRAL DIARRHEA

Viruses are the most common cause of diarrhea in children. Several groups of viruses are now recognized as affecting young children and typically occur in wintertime, when groups of children are in closest contact. Epidemics or outbreaks of diarrhea are common in schools and day-care centers and can also be passed within families. These infections are spread by hand-to-mouth contact of infected secretions (from feces), usually related to poor handwashing habits in children coupled with inadvertent contamination while at close play. Most episodes of viral diarrhea are short-lived and last from 24 hours to several days.

Viral diarrhea is mainly an inconvenience for adults but can be a serious matter in young children or debilitated elderly individuals, who potentially can become dehydrated. Viral diarrhea usually is watery, occurring in waves of eliminations, and may be associated with cramps, vomiting, low-grade fever, and body aches. High fevers are uncommon, and the stools are *never* bloody. Viruses cause diarrhea by infecting the cells lining the intestines, thus inhibiting the production of enzymes in the outermost brush border. Complex sugars (including the milk sugar lactose) are poorly absorbed and intensify the diarrhea. Antibiotics are of no use in the treatment of viral diarrhea, although proprietary medicines such as Kaopectate® (which acts by absorbing water) or Pepto-Bismol® (which may prevent viruses from binding onto intestinal cells) may be helpful. Treatment should be directed toward maintaining hydration with large amounts of fluids and salt solutions (broths, juices, and soft drinks). Hard to digest foods such as complex sugars (including milk products), fatty or greasy foods, large amounts of roughage, and seasoned foods should be avoided. The diet can be gradually advanced once the symptoms have improved. Treatment with potent antidiarrheal medications such as Lomotil®, paregoric, or Imodium® may temporarily relieve the symptoms but can prolong the natural course of the illness by slowing the elimination of the virus from the stool.

BACTERIAL DIARRHEA

Bacteria (common germs) are normal inhabitants of the colon. They are present in extraordinary numbers, up to 1,000,000,000,000 per drop (milliliter) of feces. There are over 100 different varieties of bacteria that normally live in the gut, many of which are helpful in the digestion of various foods as well as in the production of certain vitamins (e.g., folic acid and vitamin K) necessary for life.

These bacteria normally live in concert with each other and the host and even produce factors to keep harmful species of bacteria under control. It is only when this large population is disturbed by the introduction of disease-producing strains or is altered by antibiotics, that diarrhea-producing bacteria overgrow and symptoms develop.

Bacterial diarrhea typically occurs after the inadvertent ingestion of contaminated food or water. There are a large number of bacterial species (see Table 1) that are capable of producing different patterns of intestinal illnesses ranging from fevers and mild cramps with constipation to severe, bloody diarrhea. We are now able to identify most strains of disease-producing bacteria by culture of the stool from symptomatic patients. In many episodes of apparent bacterial infection, no known disease-producing strain may be isolated. In these settings we can only presume that some, as yet unidentified, ''bug'' was the culprit. This is often the case with traveler's diarrhea.

Bacterial diarrheas frequently are accompanied by higher fevers than are seen with viral illnesses, a more prolonged course lasting 7 to 14 days, and at times, bloody stools. Although many of these infections are resolved without treatment, dehydration may become a problem, and even severe prostration may occur as a result of the combination of fluid loss and fever. The dietary measures men-

Table 1. *Bacterial infections causing diarrhea*

Campylobacter
Salmonella
Shigella
E. coli (toxigenic or pathogenic strains)
Clostridium difficile (antibiotic related)
Yersinia enterocolitica
Aeromonas hydrophilia
Plesiomonas shigelloides   Rare
Edwardsiella tarda

tioned above for viral illness also are appropriate for bacterial diarrhea. Likewise, treatment with potent antidiarrheal drugs may prolong the length of the illness. The presence of more severe symptoms such as high fever or blood in the stool requires an evaluation by a physician. Depending on the specific organism and the degree of illness, the prescription of antibiotics may or may not be warranted.

PARASITES

Parasitic diarrhea is a worldwide problem, though more common in underdeveloped nations. Still, many areas of the United States supplied by untreated water are sources for infections with ameba, *Giardia*, and other, less common, parasites. Again, there is a spectrum of symptoms ranging from mild crampy diarrhea to severe bloody stools. Compared to viral or bacterial diarrhea, parasites produce a more prolonged illness, which less commonly resolves without treatment. Most individuals will develop parasitic infections after traveling to areas with untreated water (including mountain streams and well water), but they may also be contracted in industrialized cities and common vacation resorts. In many instances the infection may not fully develop for days or weeks after the initial exposure to parasites, so that an exact source of contamination may never be identified. Again, the development of diarrhea in a person who previously has had normal bowel movements should be evaluated by a physician, sooner rather than later depending on the degree of the symptoms.

TRAVELER'S DIARRHEA

After living, eating, and drinking in a particular locale, individuals develop a bacterial community within their intestines that maintains an internal balance among numerous different species of bacteria. By moving or traveling to a different location, new strains are introduced to the intestines and begin to interact with the indigenous population of bacteria. Sometimes the new strain will be incorporated in an innocuous fashion, but at other times the species will temporarily produce a flux in the bacterial population that can allow harmful bacteria to overgrow, irritate the bowel, and produce diarrhea. The resultant diarrhea may be regarded as a physiological response because the rapid transit will purge the harmful species until a new, more harmonious microbial equilibrium is achieved.

Because of the unsanitary conditions in many portions of the world, harmful bacteria are more common in underdeveloped nations, especially the tropical countries. Some species are well recognized causes of diarrhea (*Salmonella* and *Shigella*), whereas other strains are identical to bacteria that normally inhabit the intestine (*E. coli*) but have developed the ability to invade tissues or produce toxins. The latter are more difficult to identify and require special techniques not available in most hospitals or laboratories. Additionally, the lack of sanitary plumbing and water supplies may allow contamination of foods or waters by parasites such as ameba, *Giardia*, or intestinal worms. The latter may not be established for up to several weeks and thus can produce symptoms weeks after the return from foreign travel.

Protection against infectious diarrhea in foreign countries involves several relatively easy measures. The most obvious is to avoid the dirtier countries or locations. Central America, Africa, and the Middle East are notorious for harboring diarrheal infections. When traveling in these areas, you should be aware that it is the food and the water that carry the infectious agents. Therefore, the adage "don't drink the water" is protective advice. You must also be careful about exposure to tap water (used for brushing the teeth) and shower water, which should not be swallowed. Ice served in drinks also can carry harmful bacteria and should be avoided. Bottled water, boiled beverages (coffee and tea), and alcoholic beverages (wine, beer, or liquor) usually are safe. You should also be careful to avoid fresh fruits and vegetables (e.g., salads) that are washed in the contaminated water and then served. Cooked vegetables usually have been adequately sterilized unless they have been kept uneaten for long periods of time. Fruits that can be peeled are also safe.

Travelers should be particularly wary of vendors and outdoor food stands. These are the most dangerous sources of food. Restaurants and hotels provide a little more security, and if you have the opportunity to eat in a private home, this may be the best option.

Because traveler's diarrhea is such a common problem, physicians have been looking for preventive measures to obviate the need for the abovementioned precautions. No such method has yet been completely protective. Consumption of Pepto-Bismol® in fairly large quantities (an 8-oz bottle daily) will protect against most forms of diarrhea. This must be "weighed" against the disadvantage of carrying a suitcase filled with bottles of Pepto-Bismol®. Unfortunately, the tablets do not appear to be as effective in preventing diarrhea. Several antibiotics also will prevent diarrhea if taken daily. A combination sulfa tablet (Bactrim DS® or Septra DS®) taken once daily has been shown to be effective in preventing the majority of bacterial infections. Likewise, a form of tetracycline (doxycycline, Vibramycin®) has also been protective when taken daily. These drugs should not be given to everybody since they can cause allergic reactions, skin rash, or sensitivity to the sun. It is reasonable for certain individuals with chronic illnesses, including inflammatory bowel disease, to take antibiotics to prevent diarrhea. The individual circumstances should be discussed with your physician prior to the anticipated travel.

If a person develops diarrhea in a foreign country, the symptoms of a minor diarrhea (*turista*) should be distinguished from more severe dysentery. The simple variety of diarrhea usually will last several days and is more an inconvenience than a medical problem. With more severe symptoms, including bloody diarrhea or fever, you should seek medical attention. Most simple diarrheas will resolve without treatment, and the symptoms may improve with hydration (remembering to avoid fresh water or fruit drinks) as well as with the use of Pepto-Bismol® or, on occasion, Lomotil® or Imodium®. For more severe or persistent symptoms, an antibiotic should be administered under the guidance of a physician.

ANTIBIOTIC-ASSOCIATED DIARRHEA

One of the more common side effects of antibiotics is diarrhea. This may occur with virtually any antibiotic and is caused by an alteration in the normal bacterial population of the gut. When the normal equilibrium of intestinal bacteria is altered, the imbalance allows strains of bacteria that are ordinarily suppressed to grow and produce toxins that cause diarrhea. Under most circumstances, the balance will be restored on discontinuing the antibiotic. On occasion, however, the diarrhea can progress and become severe. In this situation, any individual should alert his or her physician for further advice as to the treatment of the diarrhea. In some situations an additional antibiotic may be necessary to control the harmful strain.

CHAPTER 6

Ulcerative Colitis and Proctitis

SYMPTOMS

Since the majority of individuals with ulcerative colitis and proctitis have inflammation of the surface lining of the rectum, the *cardinal symptoms* are diarrhea and bleeding from the rectum. The severity of the diarrhea relates to the extent of the large bowel involvement by the inflammatory process. When only the rectum is involved, as in proctitis, there is frequently enough surface remaining in the uninvolved colon that the usual absorption of water and formation of solid stools can be accomplished. Therefore, for some people with proctitis, the initial symptoms are bowel movements coated by blood or increased mucus accompanied by formed stools (or even constipation). These people may also notice the passage of blood or mucus alone several times during the day or night without any formed stool. When the rectum is inflamed, it may lose its ability to discriminate between solids and gas, and an individual may not be able to differentiate among the passage of gas alone, gas with small amounts of blood and mucus, or a liquid stool.

As more of the colon is involved in the inflammation, the stools may become less formed, grainy, particulate, or even watery. The stools may be associated with obvious blood and mucus, or may appear dark, port wine, or blackened in color. The number of bowel movements varies depending on diet and bowel activity. Some highly motivated individuals are able to delay moving their bowels despite frequent tenesmus (a painful spasm of the anal sphincter with an urgent desire to empty the bowel), whereas others may be unable to withhold the 20 to 30 bowel movements that may occur daily.

The diarrhea often is associated with abdominal pain, which occurs chiefly in the rectum or as a diffuse cramping that can extend across the abdomen similar to but more severe than typical "gas pain." The exact cause of the pain is not certain, but it can be related to the inflammation irritating pain receptors in the muscles of the bowel wall, excessive contraction and spasms of the bowel musculature, and the accentuated irritability of the bowel.

When the inflammation is more severe or extensive, these symptoms may be accompanied by fever ranging from 99°–100°F to 104°F. The fever may be intermittent or persistent. Weight loss occurs because individuals experience less diarrhea when they eat less. A reduction in diet also may improve the abdominal pain, and over a period of weeks, the individual learns to control symptoms by decreasing food intake. When severe, the crampy abdominal pain and diarrhea may be associated with vomiting and may lead to dehydration and prostration.

DIAGNOSIS

The diagnosis of ulcerative colitis or proctitis is first and foremost based on the exclusion of known forms of diarrhea. Cultures of the stool must be obtained to identify potential bacterial and other infectious diarrhea. Examining the rectum with a proctoscope (a short lighted tube) demonstrates typical changes of the lining surface of the rectum. These changes include tiny confluent ulcerations with or without active bleeding and pus. When the inflammation is limited to the rectum, the physician will be able to maneuver the proctoscope beyond the area of inflammation to normal colon mucosa. The proctoscopic examination is usually more embarrassing than painful and is well tolerated by the great majority of our patients when performed in a gentle and discreet manner.

Another means of examining the rectum and sigmoid colon is by a flexible sigmoidoscope, which is a slightly longer tube than a proctoscope and has the advantages of (a) being flexible so that it can bend in all directions and even form a loop on itself, (b) having an extremely bright light source allowing the examiner to see the mucosa in a magnified view, and (c) because of new technology, allowing smaller biopsies to be obtained through this endoscope. The flexible sigmoidoscope is long enough to reach the splenic flexure of the colon in many patients and hence allows the physician to examine above the area of inflammation in those patients with only distal (left-sided) colitis. To do so requires more preparation (such as enemas), so that a simple proctoscopic examination is often preferred as a first diagnostic test.

The colonoscope is an even longer flexible tube that is otherwise the same as a flexible sigmoidoscope and is capable of reaching the full length of the colon and even into the terminal ileum. We perform this examination with a combination of analgesia (pain medication) and sedative. These premedications are given because of the length of time it takes to examine the colon (approximately 30 minutes) as well as to improve some of the cramping that is associated with stretching of the colon by the scope itself. This examination is well tolerated by the vast majority of patients who are kept comfortable by the medication and offered considerate assistance. As might be expected, such a complete and thorough examination requires a more vigorous preparation including a liquid diet over several days as well as laxatives and/or enemas.

When direct examination is not feasible, or if a permanent record is important, X-ray studies of the colon also may document the diagnosis of ulcerative colitis. Since only the lining of the colon is affected in this condition, excellent preparation of the colon is important so the physician will be able to visualize subtle findings. We prefer a 2-day preparation of clear liquids. During this time, the patient is also given a laxative to further clear the colon of fecal material, which might otherwise obscure the fine details of the mucosa. We also perform this X-ray examination, the barium enema, with a combination of air and barium (double-contrast or air-contrast barium enema) in order to record the often subtle changes involving the colonic surface. Again, when this examination is performed by a team of experienced and compassionate radiologists and technicians, it usually can be accomplished without sedation and with only a minimal degree of discomfort to the patient. When performed well, the examination can define very slight alterations along the lining of the colon and can be used as a basis of comparison for future examinations.

In difficult cases when cultures are negative and the typical X-ray or endoscopic (proctoscopic or colonoscopic) findings are in-conclusive, a biopsy of the colon may be obtained through either the proctoscope or the flexible endoscopes. The biopsy consists of removing a pinch of tissue from the superficial layer of the colon, and since there are no pain fibers in this portion, the procedure is completely painless. Also, since it is a shallow sample, there is only rarely significant bleeding from the biopsy site. When examined under the microscope, the tissue sample usually will demonstrate typical features of ulcerative colitis, although at times even the biopsy findings may not be entirely conclusive.

Unfortunately, there are no specific laboratory findings specific for ulcerative colitis or, for that matter, Crohn's disease. There is no specific blood test that will identify these diseases individually, nor is there a specific group of diagnostic blood tests. In the future, it may be possible to label an individual's own blood cells with a radioactive chemical to observe where these blood cells migrate within the bowel and, hence, define the areas of inflammation. However, as yet this is only an experimental tool. In the future, a specific blood or pathologic marker may be identified that will help toward the definite diagnosis of inflammatory bowel disease. For the moment, the diagnosis depends on a well-informed physician who is able to recognize the features compatible with this illness and who will be able to interpret the various X-rays and endoscopic findings accurately.

INTESTINAL COMPLICATIONS

The complications of ulcerative colitis and proctitis include those that occur within the bowel (intestinal) and those that occur outside of the bowel (extraintestinal).

The most common intestinal complication of ulcerative colitis is *hemorrhage* or excessive bleeding. The exact nature of the bleeding in ulcerative colitis is not always clear. When an observer wipes the mucosa with a cotton swab through an endoscope, there frequently is oozing of blood from the colon tissue (friability). Likewise, the passage of a stool will often induce bleeding around the stool. As the inflammation progresses and becomes more extensive, the entire bowel lining may become weepy and persistently ooze blood. In rare instances, bleeding can become profuse and persistent. Usually this responds to medical treatment (see Treatment section). However, in rare instances, the hemorrhage is so extensive that an emergency operation is required to remove the colon (colectomy).

A second emergency complication of ulcerative colitis occurs in rare situations when colonic motor activity ceases and the large intestine expands to several times its normal diameter. This condition is known as *toxic megacolon* and frequently is associated with very severe symptoms including fever, abdominal pain, toxic state, and prostration. This is a rare but most serious complication of ulcerative colitis. When the colon dilates, the entire thickness of the bowel becomes inflamed and weakened and at some points becomes as thin as wet toilet paper. If there is not an immediate response (within hours) to medical therapy, then surgical removal of the colon is a necessity to prevent perforation of the colon and the leakage of infected bowel contents into the abdominal cavity. At times, the colon will have become so fragile that by the time the surgeon operates it will literally fall apart in his hands. Fortunately, this is a rare occurrence in ulcerative colitis.

In addition to the immediate complications described above, chronic or longstanding ulcerative colitis can produce unique problems. One such complication is a *stricture,* or narrowing, of the colon that may develop after many years of disease. This narrowing results from thickening of the muscular layers of the colon and can limit the diameter quite significantly, so that bowel movements may be altered. Rarely, however, does the lumen of the intestine narrow so much that a complete blockage (obstruction) ensues. Although these strictures usually are benign and of no consequence, the major difficulty they pose is discriminating between a benign stricture and a cancer, which may appear similar.

Many patients are already aware that longstanding ulcerative colitis can impose an increased risk of developing cancer of the large intestine. As physicians have become more cognizant of this potential complication, more careful observations of the patterns of malignancies in ulcerative colitis have led to advances in the detection and early therapy for these cancers.

Rarely do such cancers develop before ulcerative colitis has been present for at least 10 years. After the first decade, there is approximately a 10% risk of developing a malignancy for each decade of disease. For instance, after a 30-year course of ulcerative colitis, there is approximately a 30% risk or one-in-three chance of developing a cancer. When a cancer does develop, it behaves in the same way as any colon cancer. It is now known that these tumors arise as small growths or polyps that enlarge slowly. At first, the growth does not extend below the mucosal or superficial layer of the intestinal wall, and at this point it is *totally curable* by removal. If the tumor extends into the deeper layers or through the muscle layers of the colon wall, there is a greater risk that cells from the tumor will invade the bloodstream or lymphatic vessels. Although it may take up to several years for a tumor to become large enough to invade the muscle layers, once it has progressed into the lymphatic system, it is much more difficult to treat. From the lymphatic vessels, the tumor will usually spread (metastasize) into lymph nodes within the abdomen, and the liver. Once the tumor has spread into distant nodes or the liver, it is rarely curable, although chemotherapy techniques are improving, and there is great hope for the future.

One of the most important medical developments has been the use of colonoscopy in screening patients with ulcerative colitis for cancer. Our understanding of how cancer develops has been greatly advanced by the observation that tumors do not develop *de novo* from normal or even inflamed colon. Instead, the cells lining the mucosa begin to change their appearance and become dysplastic (have the potential for altered growth). Dysplastic cells may undergo even more atypical changes before they become malignant and eventually develop into a tumor that has the potential to invade and destroy distant tissues. We recently have recognized different gradations of dysplasia and are just beginning to comprehend their clinical significance.

After a patient has had ulcerative colitis for more than 5 or 10 years, we recommend that he or she undergo complete colonoscopic examinations at regular intervals (at least every 2 years). At the time of the colonoscopy, any area of the colon that looks abnormal will be biopsied, and additional random samples are taken along the length of the colon. We then examine this tissue under the microscope to look for changes of dysplasia. When there is low-grade or only mild dysplasia, we usually recommend follow-up. If we suspect that the dysplastic changes are of a high grade or the cells are extremely abnormal, then the risk of developing a cancer becomes imminent, and we believe that if this finding is confirmed, it is an indication for removing the entire colon.

Medical investigators are continuing to try to ascertain the colonic events that lead to cancer. The development of a malignancy in ulcerative colitis seems to depend on at least two factors. We know that patients whose entire colon is involved are more likely to develop a cancer than patients with proctitis or left-sided colitis, although in the latter instance, the tumor may be delayed in its appearance by 10 years or longer. The other factor is the length of time an individual has had the disease. Whether there are other factors leading to the development of a malignancy such as a family history of colon cancer, the degree of inflammation, any medical treatment, or other as yet undetermined factors such as the geographic environment (e.g., United States) are questions that remain to be answered.

A final comment about cancer in ulcerative colitis is that the most important determinant for a good outcome, as with any cancer, is early detection. If the cancers are detected when they are small and have not yet invaded the bowel wall, they are almost always completely curable. We are even more comfortable when we can detect the imminent development of a malignancy by finding severe dysplasia. Under these circumstances, the complete removal of the colon and rectum (proctocolectomy) will obviate the risk of developing a colon cancer in the future. Many patients with a long history of quiet and uncomplicated ulcerative colitis ask if a less drastic operation such as partial colectomy (leaving the rectum in place, thus preserving rectal and anal function) might be considered. Although this is a possibility, we do not recommend leaving any of the colon behind except in unusual individual circumstances. If a partial colectomy is performed leaving the rectal tissue within the colon, the remaining mucosa is still vulnerable and at continued risk of developing cancer. As long as any colonic tissue remains, we believe that continued screening is indicated on a regular basis. If significant dysplasia or a malignancy is found, then another operation to remove the rectum should be performed.

EXTRAINTESTINAL COMPLICATIONS

Numerous potential complications of ulcerative colitis do not involve the intestinal tract. The most frequent arises directly from rectal bleeding and is anemia (low red blood cell count). The anemia is usually caused by a deficiency of iron, which is lost from the body in the form of blood in greater amounts than are manufactured by the body. The treatment of iron deficiency anemia consists of improving the abdominal inflammation as well as replacing the iron. The iron that is lost can be replaced by blood transfusion, administration of iron tablets, or injection of iron compounds into either the muscles or by infusion into a vein.

For patients who tolerate iron replacement by mouth, this is the preferred method. For patients who are still symptomatic with cramping or diarrhea, we find that iron tablets often irritate the digestive tract. We then provide the iron supplements in the form of a blood transfusion or by injection. Intramuscular injection of iron requires a deep muscular penetration, which is often painful and will stain the skin a dark blue-brown color. Hence, we are beginning to administer intravenous (i.v.) iron more frequently. A small test dose is initially dripped in to the vein to insure that there are no allergic reactions. The full replacement is then given as an i.v. drip over several hours. The latter method is usually well tolerated, although some people may develop an allergic reaction such as wheezing, swollen lips, or a skin rash. A few individuals develop a delayed reaction similar to the "flu" with fever and muscle or joint aches that develop 1 or 2 days after the iron infusion has been completed. This is an uncommon and unique side effect of intravenous iron and occurs after a large dose has been administered. The symptoms may linger for a day or two but then disappear without any complications. It is not a true allergic reaction, and iron has been given on subsequent occasions to individuals who have had these symptoms.

Another form of anemia relates to sulfasalazine (Azulfidine®) treatment. Sulfasalazine is known to interfere with the absorption of folic acid from food. Folic acid is a necessary vitamin for the production of blood cells. When individuals become deficient in folic acid, an underproduction of blood cells and anemia can ensue, and the red blood cells increase in size. The simplest method of preventing this effect of sulfasalazine is to replace the folic acid with a 1-mg tablet taken daily with the sulfasalazine. A folic acid deficiency is treated by doubling the dosage of folic acid to 2 mg daily. Sulfasalazine also has been associated with less common forms of anemia in which the red blood cells actually break apart (hemolytic anemia). In rare individuals who are deficient in a particular enzyme (G-6-PD) that normally protects the red blood cells, the addition of sulfasalazine may produce increased destruction of blood cells, leading to anemia. This form of anemia will usually occur shortly after beginning the drug and may present as jaundice (yellowing of the skin and eyes). It is corrected by discontinuing the medication.

Vitamin deficiencies other than folic acid deficiency can occur in ulcerative colitis if an individual restricts the diet in order to control symptoms. Although the vitamin deficiency can be severe, it is usually only mild and can be avoided in the great majority of patients by treating the individual's symptoms to the point that he or she is able to eat a more regular diet. We usually recommend a single multiple vitamin for any patient with prolonged symptoms of diarrhea.

Other potential complications are less directly related to the loss of compounds from the inflamed bowel. Several disorders of the liver and gallbladder have been recognized as occurring more frequently in inflammatory bowel disease. A mild inflammatory condition of the liver, termed *pericholangitis*, can occur in ulcerative colitis in up to 50% of individuals. The inflammation is possibly caused by bacteria that enter the bloodstream in the inflamed colon and are subsequently filtered in the liver. Although the exact cause of pericholangitis has not been identified, it is felt that the increased load of bacteria to the liver incites an inflammatory reaction in the smaller bile passages (ducts). This inflammation does not appear to progress to a destructive form of liver disease and usually is asymptomatic, manifesting only as a mild abnormality in blood tests of liver function.

In a very few individuals with ulcerative colitis, there is a much more severe inflammation around the bile ducts called sclerosing cholangitis. This is a progressive form of liver damage in which the bile ducts may become damaged enough to impair the flow of bile and can lead to chronic liver failure. Fortunately, the latter disease is extremely uncommon.

Many individuals with inflammatory bowel disease develop muscular or skeletal symptoms at one point or another during their illness, usually when the bowel disease is in a period of activity. The cause of these symptoms is unknown, but it is felt by many of us to be bacteria or bacterial products that gain entry into the bloodstream through the injured gut and are attacked there by antibodies to form complexes with the foreign antigenic material. These antibody–antigen complexes are then filtered in various locations throughout the body, often by the lining membrane of joints. In the joint membranes, the complexes are further metabolized, and they induce an inflammatory response, causing arthritis with joint redness, swelling, and fluid accumulation. The arthritis associated with ulcerative colitis typically occurs in the large joints of the lower limbs, especially the knees and ankles, but may also be present in the hips, elbows, wrists, or almost any joint. The arthritis is rarely crippling or progressive and usually improves as the bowel disease improves. For particularly troublesome symptoms, a number of medications may be prescribed to improve the arthritis. Most of these drugs are related to aspirin and are effective in treating the arthritis. Care must be used in prescribing these medications because of potential side effects of stomach irritation or ulcers as well as the enhanced propensity for bleeding. The latter results from impairment in the function of platelets (a type of blood cell necessary for blood to clot).

More unusual forms of arthritis also have been associated with inflammatory bowel disease that involve the spine and pelvis. *Sacroiliitis* and *ankylosing spondylitis* are inflammatory diseases of the sacroiliac joints in the pelvis and spine, respectively, that occur most frequently in individuals with a particular genetic background and who possess a specific blood antigen (HLA-B27). Sacroiliitis is an inflammatory condition of the sacroiliac joint in the pelvis and causes low back pain. Ankylosing spondylitis is a similar inflammatory condition of the lower spine and may evolve into a stiffening and straightening of the back with an eventual fusion or gluing of the vertebrae so that an affected individual would not be able to bend his or her spine when leaning over. Although these conditions occur infrequently in ulcerative colitis (fewer than 5% of individuals), those who have HLA-B27 marker are much more susceptible to these forms of arthritis. They are treated with a combination of exercises to improve flexibility and antiinflammatory medications.

A variety of skin rashes occur in the setting of ulcerative colitis. *Erythema nodosum* may develop in up to 10% of people with ulcerative colitis and presents as tender nodules that occur frequently over the legs and shins of women much more frequently than men. The nodules, or bumps, are raised, red or reddish-blue, warm, and tender and usually fade over time and occur more commonly when the bowel symptoms are active. *Pyoderma gangrenosum* is a much less common but serious skin lesion that occurs as an ulceration also appearing most frequently on the legs, especially after bumping or bruising. The condition may be a deep and painful ulcerating sore that is difficult to treat and should receive immediate medical attention. Therapy involves intensive local therapy of the skin with corticosteroid cream and topical antibiotics in addition to controlling the underlying disease.

Numerous nonspecific skin rashes also may occur in patients with ulcerative colitis, including eczema, psoriasis, and hives, which may be attributed to the bowel inflammation or a reaction to the drug used in treating the colitis. They are usually neither progressive nor severe.

Several eye problems are also associated with ulcerative colitis. Inflammation can occur (iritis, uveitis) that usually causes pain and redness of the eye and can be associated with other skin manifestations. These problems are usually improved with corticosteroid drops to the eye but require the attention of a physician.

URINARY COMPLICATIONS

There is an increased tendency toward the development of kidney stones in ulcerative colitis, although the exact mechanism has yet to be determined. It is likely that the increased metabolism evoked by the ongoing inflammatory process increases the body's production of uric acid, which, when concentrated in the urine, can form the beginning of a stone. Dehydration also plays a part in the formation of kidney stones related to ulcerative colitis, and an adequate fluid intake, especially in cases of diarrhea, should be maintained.

MISCELLANEOUS DISORDERS

A variety of other less frequent complications can occur during the course of ulcerative colitis. Blood clots are seen more frequently and are usually related to the increased production of clotting proteins that is induced by the inflammation. Growth retardation may also occur in children with ulcerative colitis and may be related to poor nutrition as well as to the use of corticosteroids (see Chapter 12). The prognosis for reaching normal height is usually good, and growth spurts typically coincide with improvements of the inflammatory process.

Infertility also has been seen in some men with ulcerative colitis being treated with sulfasalazine. This is related to alterations in the sperm in some individuals on this medication. Some effects on the sperm may be secondary to impairment of folic acid absorption by the sulfasalazine, and we usually prescribe additional folic acid for anybody taking this drug. Problems of infertility also may be related to the chronic illness or to treatment with corticosteroids but are relatively uncommon. Aside from irregular or absent menstruation in females with ulcerative colitis, women are fertile, can become pregnant, and will usually carry normal children. It is best to undertake pregnancy when the illness has been well controlled. It should also be mentioned that neither colectomy nor ileostomy will impair either sexual function or the ability to carry children to a normal delivery.

TREATMENT

Because ulcerative colitis is limited to the colon, there is a singular curative treatment. Unfortunately, this involves surgical removal of the entire colon and rectum. Short of this radical cure, ulcerative colitis is a chronic process that can be treated medically but often has a variable course of remissions and exacerbations.

We believe in various stages of therapy for ulcerative colitis depending on the symptoms and the extent of the inflammatory process. For individuals with no rectal bleeding but only mild diarrhea, dietary restrictions alone may improve the symptoms. A low-residue diet, avoiding unrefined roughage in the form of seeds, nuts, corn, and raw fruits and vegetables in favor of cooked, canned, or peeled fruits and vegetables, is a first line of defense against the frequent bowel movements. Individuals who have symptoms from drinking milk should avoid milk products or ingest them in association with a product (LactAid® or Lactrase™) to predigest the milk sugar lactose.

For abdominal cramps or diarrhea not responsive to dietary alterations alone, adding an antispasmodic (e.g., tincture of belladonna or Bentyl®) or an antispasmodic in addition to a mild sedative (e.g., Donnatal®, Librax®, Combid®) may be helpful. When looser stools are frequent, then an antidiarrheal preparation such as Lomotil® or Imodium® may be used. However, in severe cases of colitis associated with bloody diarrhea, fevers, or abdominal pain, these medications should be used only under the careful supervision of a physician since they can potentiate the development of a toxic dilatation of the colon.

Sulfasalazine (Azulfidine®) is a combination of two medications, a sulfonamide antibiotic (sulfapyridine) attached to a unique salicylate [5-aminosalicylic acid (5-ASA)] by a chemical bond. When taken orally very little of the medication is absorbed, and when the drug reaches the colon, bacteria split the medication into its two components. The sulfapyridine is absorbed into the bloodstream from the bowel and is excreted by the kidney. Recent studies have shown that the sulfapyridine, a weak antibacterial drug, has no influence on the inflamed bowel yet accounts for the majority of the side effects of sulfasalazine including headache, nausea, and the majority of allergic reactions (skin rash, fever, hepatitis). The 5-ASA, a derivative of aspirin, remains within the colon and appears to account for the majority of the beneficial antiinflammatory effects.

Sulfasalazine is the most effective medication to date for maintaining a remission in ulcerative colitis. The drug is used to treat mild to moderate symptoms of ulcerative colitis and should be maintained for up to several years after the last episode of colitis. Unfortunately, many people develop side effects or are unable to tolerate the drug, and a few individuals are allergic to the medication. As we begin to understand more about this unique drug, it appears that the majority of the side effects are caused by the sulfa component, and several drug companies are currently attempting to produce an active compound without the sulfa. 5-Aminosalicylic acid enemas have been used effectively in Europe, and certain similar products in oral or enema form are currently being tested in the United States and abroad.

Cortisone and its derivatives (steroids) are the most potent antiinflammatory drugs available for the treatment of ulcerative colitis. For mild symptoms of colitis involving only the left colon, enema preparations of hydrocortisone (Cortenema®), methylprednisolone (Medrol®), or hydrocortisone-impregnated foam (Cortifoam®) may be used to improve the symptoms of rectal urgency, pain, and bleeding. When symptoms of colitis are more severe or extensive, these medications may be administered in an oral form or by intramuscular or intravenous injection, depending on the setting. ACTH is a hormone that induces the adrenal gland to produce high levels of cortisone, with similar beneficial effects.

The corticosteroid preparations have many beneficial as well as undesirable effects. The drugs should not be taken and, most certainly, should not be discontinued without the knowledge of your physician. (Of course, this is true for all medications, not just corticosteroids.)

At the present time there is only one surgical procedure that should be considered in ulcerative colitis. This is a conservative operation consisting of the removal of the entire colon and rectum with the formation of an *ileostomy*. Experimental methods are currently being investigated involving either an internal pouch underneath the abdominal wall that can be emptied through a nipple valve in the skin or the formation of a direct connection between the ileum to the anus after stripping off the rectal lining. These should be considered experimental methods, and we do not recommend them for the typical patient. We feel that these should be used only in medical centers where active investigation regarding the physiology, complication rate, and outcome of these procedures is being pursued.

PROGNOSIS

The long-term outcome of ulcerative colitis depends on many factors including the location of the inflammatory reaction, the extent of inflammation (mild versus severe), the age at which colitis develops, the total length of time that one has had colitis, and the complications that have ensued. When ulcerative colitis is limited to the rectum, as with proctitis, the condition is more often inconvenient, irritating, and troublesome than severe or life threatening. On the other hand, when ulcerative colitis presents with a severe first episode accompanied by debilitating symptoms requiring hospitalization, a colectomy is more often necessary.

Depending on the patient's and physician's perseverance with medical therapy, surgery for ulcerative colitis may be required in 15 to 50% of individuals; our own figure approximates 20 to 25%. The major risk of requiring a colectomy usually is during the first few years of the disease, and children and adolescents who develop colitis have a greater risk of requiring a colectomy because colitis is more severe in this group, and the susceptibility to growth retardation is, at times, another reason for surgery. Among all individuals who undergo a colectomy, there is approximately a one-in-four chance that additional surgery for mechanical conditions such as revision of the ileostomy or small hernias (a weakness in the abdominal wall muscle) or an intestinal obstruction may be required.

The risk of cancer in the course of ulcerative colitis has been discussed. As screening techniques such as colonoscopy and biopsy of the colon looking for dysplasia become more routine, we believe that this risk will be lessened, although possibly at the expense of additional surgical procedures.

The survival of patients with ulcerative colitis naturally depends on the severity of the illness. There is an increased risk of severe complications during the first several years of the disease, after which the survival of individuals with ulcerative colitis seems to parallel that of the general public. Patients who develop ulcerative colitis after the age of 50 tend to have a worse prognosis than younger patients. This may be related to other concomitant medical problems besides the ulcerative colitis.

In discussing the prognosis, it is important to consider the quality of life of individuals afflicted with this chronic disease. Most individuals with ulcerative colitis lead an entirely normal life except for more frequent outpatient hospital visits. Most people with colitis consider their quality of life as "good to fair," and only a small proportion as "poor." Patients with ulcerative colitis have comparable marital status, frequency of severe family or sexual problems, leisure activities, and physical and earning capacities as people without the illness. Although there are individuals with distinct problems related to ulcerative colitis who will require individual or family counseling (see Chapter 11), this group of individuals, as a whole, seems to adapt well to the condition and do not appear to suffer excessive social or professional disabilities.

CHAPTER 7

Crohn's Disease

SYMPTOMS

Crohn's disease can involve any portion of the gastrointestinal tract from the mouth to the anus. Hence, the symptoms of any individual will depend on the location of the inflammatory process as well as on the nonintestinal complications unique to Crohn's disease.

Whereas rectal bleeding is most common in ulcerative colitis, it is a less frequent manifestation of Crohn's disease. On the other hand, diarrhea and cramping abdominal pain are more typical and occur in the majority of individuals. Constipation is a rare but occasional symptom. Fever, which may be intermittent and associated with chills or night sweats, is a subtle symptom of Crohn's disease. Weight loss is also a commonly associated feature, which may be related to decreased appetite, altered sensation of taste, or decreased food consumption in order to prevent symptoms.

In the upper digestive tract, painless ulcerations of the mouth, lips, throat, and voice box may precede or accompany flare-ups of the intestinal disease. Inflammation can occur in the esophagus, causing heartburn or pain with swallowing. In the stomach, Crohn's disease is usually without symptoms but may cause nausea, vomiting, or upper abdominal pain. In the duodenum, active Crohn's disease is virtually indistinguishable from a peptic ulcer, with symptoms of burning abdominal pain, nausea, and vomiting.

More typically, Crohn's disease affects the small intestine, producing symptoms of lower abdominal pain that may be associated with cramps, bloating, and vomiting if the bowel becomes partially blocked. Inflammation may involve several loops of bowel, which become thickened and adherent, producing a tender abdominal mass (swelling), most typically in the lower right portion of the abdomen. Malabsorption of food products causes diarrhea and weight loss. When the appendix is involved, the condition mimics appendicitis with severe abdominal pain, nausea, vomiting, and fever and necessitates operation.

With involvement of the colon, the symptoms of Crohn's disease may be virtually indistinguishable from those of ulcerative colitis. Diarrhea (with or without blood), crampy pain, and rectal discomforts are common. Rectal pain may be present if the lower portions of the colon are inflamed. Thin or ribbon-like stools may occur if the rectum is narrowed or if a stricture is present.

Some unique features of Crohn's disease help to distinguish this process from ulcerative colitis. Crohn's disease often spares the rectum but involves the anus with large, painful, protuberant hemorrhoids and fissures. Fistulas in and around the anal area are common and are the source of a discharge consisting of mucus, blood, and feces. Such fistulas may penentrate adjacent structures such as the genital tract in women, producing a rectal–vaginal fistula. Abscesses around the anus and buttocks also are more frequent in Crohn's disease and at times require surgical incisions to drain pus (Fig. 6).

DIAGNOSIS

The diagnosis of Crohn's disease is made difficult because of the wide spectrum of symptoms and the numerous potential areas of bowel involvement. At times, the initial manifestations are so insidious that the physician may not even consider a bowel disorder. The early symptoms may be so subtle as to be attributed erroneously to more commonly encountered conditions such as viral infections, appendicitis, and a "nervous stomach."

The definite diagnosis of Crohn's disease is based on a combination of symptoms, laboratory findings, X-rays, and biopsies. The location of the disease will determine the initial approach and the combination of methods that will be utilized to confirm the diagnosis.

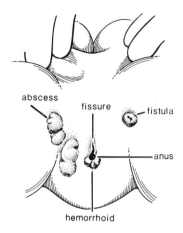

FIG. 6. Perianal Crohn's disease.

The most commonly involved area of the bowel in Crohn's disease is the terminal ileum. The initial symptoms may be as subtle as low-grade fever and/or as dramatic as severe abdominal pain mimicking acute appendicitis or complete blockage of the intestines. Eventually, most individuals will develop lower abdominal pain, often localized to the right side and accompanied by diarrhea. Progressive constipation will occasionally occur in the presence of a partial blockage of the intestines. Any of the other intestinal or inflammatory symptoms previously mentioned may also occur in association with nonintestinal complications to be discussed later.

The ileum is not easy to investigate because of the great length of bowel above and below this segment that needs to be traversed in order to visualize it either by X-ray or by an endoscope. Most commonly, this is accomplished by an "upper GI" X-ray, for which the patient swallows barium and then, by X-ray, its transit down the length of the small intestine is observed. During this examination the radiologist (a physician skilled in performing X-rays) will need to position the patient on the X-ray table carefully to obtain optimal views of this segment of small intestine. Frequently, it is necessary to take multiple X-rays, and at times this requires compression of the abdomen to separate loops of bowel so that individual segments may be scrutinized. The last portion of the ileum also may be visualized during a barium enema if the barium can be refluxed back from the colon into the ileum. This may provide a clue that the small intestine is involved, in which case a small intestine X-ray should then be performed. These examinations preferably are not performed on the same day, since it is important to visualize each segment of bowel most carefully to document the extent of the inflammatory process completely. A colonoscopic examination also may be performed when, under the best of circumstances, the colonoscope is able to be maneuvered through the ileocecal valve into the terminal ileum, where biopsies can be obtained.

Other areas of the small intestine also are evaluated by means of upper GI barium X-rays, which may be performed using two different techniques. The routine small bowel X-ray is performed as described earlier by having the patient swallow the barium. In this situation, the esophagus and stomach are also examined. As the barium empties from the stomach, the entirety of the small intestine is observed as the column of barium passes down, providing an acceptable examination in most circumstances. In some situations it is necessary to control the flow of barium to better visualize particular segments of the small bowel. For instance, at times the stomach may not empty in an optimum fashion to allow an adequate examination, or, alternatively, the stomach may empty too rapidly, and the area of interest is rapidly obscured by an overflow of barium. A special form of small intestinal X-ray, an enteroclysis, then may be preferred. For this examination, a small tube must be passed through the nose and swallowed. The tube is advanced through the esophagus and stomach into the duodenum and first portion of the small intestine, and barium is then administered through the tube in a controlled fashion so that the appropriate areas of the small intestine can be examined. When this examination is performed by an experienced radiologist, it is well tolerated and allows the most critical and definitive inspection of the small intestine.

When the colon is involved by Crohn's disease, a colonoscopic examination similar to that described for ulcerative colitis may be performed. At colonoscopy, biopsies are taken along the length of the colon, and the distribution, appearance, and focal nature of the Crohn's disease, differentiating it from ulcerative colitis, can be ascertained. Skipped areas of inflammation may be visualized and biopsied through the colonoscope, documenting both gross ulceration and microscopic involvement with typical pathologic features. One such feature is the granuloma. However, this is not a requisite for the diagnosis of Crohn's disease, for in the absence of granulomas on the biopsy specimens, the focal pattern of Crohn's disease is unlike the uniform distribution of inflammation seen in ulcerative colitis.

Crohn's disease affecting the esophagus, stomach, or duodenum may be evaluated by a combination of X-rays of the stomach and upper GI endoscopy (gastroscopy). The barium swallow is performed as described earlier except that care is taken to obtain X-ray views of the barium as it is swallowed together with special views of the stomach.

Upper intestinal endoscopy uses an endoscope similar to the colonoscope except for a shorter length and smaller diameter. The scope is quite flexible and is easy to swallow, allowing a magnified view for the physician as well as the opportunity to obtain biopsy specimens. At our institution, patients are given medication before the procedure to allow them to relax as well as an intravenous sedative during the endoscopy so that they are awake, yet completely comfortable. The medication has some amnesia effect, and many patients do not remember the examination. Additionally, the throat is numbed so that the patients will have no trouble swallowing the scope. Once the patient is comfortable, he or she is asked to swallow the scope, which is then passed into the esophagus. Patients are able to breath quite freely around the scope as it is advanced into the stomach. A small amount of air is injected to distend the stomach so that it may be completely examined, and then the instrument is advanced through the stomach into the duodenum. Biopsies may be taken, which are again painless. There are relatively few complications of this procedure when performed by an experienced examiner since the scope is quite flexible and soft. When difficulties do arise, they are more often the result of adverse reactions to the medication given to sedate the patient than of the procedure itself.

At times, a physician will see a patient with the rapid onset of lower abdominal pain that cannot be distinguished from appendicitis. These individuals may be taken to the operating room where at surgery the doctor may be surprised to find the appendix normal, but instead, the last portion of the ileum or abdominal lymph nodes inflamed. Under these circumstances, the surgeon may or may not remove the appendix but will likely take a biopsy of an inflamed lymph node to confirm the presence of Crohn's disease. The abdominal wall is then closed, and the patient can be started on medical therapy.

As with ulcerative colitis, it is important to exclude infections as a cause of the symptoms in patients with diarrhea. Cultures of the stool should be obtained as well as a microscopic examination of the feces. The demonstration of white blood cells in the stool would suggest an inflammatory process, but only cultures can exclude an associated infectious process.

Blood tests will not confirm the diagnosis of Crohn's disease but may support the doctor's suspicion. The presence of anemia, an elevated white blood cell count, increase in the sedimentation rate (a general indication of an inflammatory process occurring in the body), low serum proteins, a depressed cholesterol level (suggesting that the patient may be malabsorbing nutrients), and mild abnormalities in liver function tests all may be identified in active Crohn's disease.

When all of the above are considered, and other forms of bowel disease have been excluded, then a tentative diagnosis of Crohn's is appropriate. Even then, the doctor must maintain a persistent skepticism regarding the diagnosis during the initial stages of treatment and must keep an open mind at times of symptomatic flare-ups to exclude all curable (infectious) forms of inflammatory bowel disease.

INTESTINAL COMPLICATIONS

As with ulcerative colitis, massive hemorrhage (bleeding) may also complicate Crohn's disease. Although less common in Crohn's disease, extensive bleeding may occur from ulcerations in the colon or small intestine. When the bleeding originates from the colon, the stool will usually contain bright red blood. If the bleeding originates in the small intestine, there may be a combination of bright red blood accompanied by partially digested blood, which may impart a reddish-brown or even black color to the stool. Black, tarry stools are a symptom of upper intestinal bleeding, which must be distinguished from the greenish-black or black color that occurs when individuals take iron as a mineral supplement. Bright red color in the stool may occasionally be caused by innocuous chemicals present in beets and red food dyes.

Toxic dilation of the intestines may also occur as an unusual complication of Crohn's disease of the colon and is just as serious as when it develops in ulcerative colitis. The development of severe abdominal pain, fever, and abdominal tenderness associated with prostration, and the passage of small amounts of liquid and usually bloody stools may herald this extremely serious condition, which requires urgent medical attention. If there is not a rapid response to treatment, which includes complete bed rest, nothing by mouth, and usually a nasogastric tube to alleviate abdominal distension as well as fluids, antibiotics, and steroids, then an operation is mandatory.

Because of the nature of inflammation in Crohn's disease, which extends through all of the layers of the intestinal wall, strictures may occur with healing (Fig. 7). These are different from the strictures encountered in ulcerative colitis in that the stricture of Crohn's disease consists of fibrous or scar tissue rather than an increase in the thickness of the intestinal muscle. Because of the nature of the scarring, these strictures are much less distensible and, more commonly, will cause an obstruction or complete blockage of the passage of stool contents. The strictures can occur anywhere in the intestinal tract, although their presence in the esophagus and stomach is rare. In the small intestine, they present as a gradual increase in abdominal pain, which is made worse by eating. Ingestion of food increases intestinal peristalsis and, with a narrowing in the bowel, the peristaltic waves further increase pressures as the intestinal contents are forced through the narrowing. These conditions produce cramps, bloating, abdominal distention (swelling), and

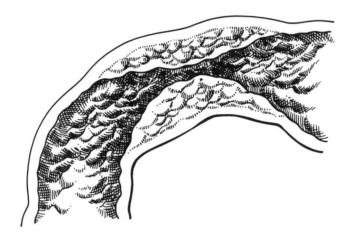

FIG. 7. Crohn's disease stricture.

may cause high-pitched abdominal bowel sounds or gurgles as the material is squeezed through the narrowed segment of bowel.

If the narrowing becomes extremely small, then a partial blockage or even complete obstruction of the intestinal flow may occur. In the latter instance, the above symptoms may be associated with progressive nausea and vomiting. At first the vomited material may consist of partially digested food, later bile or greenish intestinal contents, and finally feculent material. This may lead to dehydration if the individual is unable to hold down enough fluids, in which case the patient should certainly seek medical attention.

Strictures of the colon in Crohn's disease are generally considered to be an anticipated feature of the disease rather than a complication. The symptoms may be a gradual alteration in stool quality, initially manifested as thin ribbon-like stools with increasing constipation, which may then progress to the passage of only liquid stools. This occurs because solid material will no longer pass through the narrow area, and eventually only liquid stool is capable of traversing the diminished diameter of the lumen. Obstruction can occur and is more likely if undigested food such as nuts or seeds, or globules of fiber (e.g., celery) block the entrance to the stricture, preventing material from passing through. This is one reason why patients with Crohn's disease should avoid difficult to digest roughage.

Because benign strictures are so common in Crohn's disease, the concern about an associated cancer is not as compelling as in ulcerative colitis. These strictures may, however, be an indication for surgery if obstructions or partial obstructions continue to occur. In this setting, a limited operation to remove the stricture and the adjacent inflammatory reaction may bring symptomatic relief. On the other hand, in longstanding Crohn's disease, strictures make it difficult to screen for cancer because a colonoscope will be unable to fully visualize the colon.

Abdominal abscesses and fistulas are characteristic of Crohn's disease. They should be considered as an extension of the same pathologic process, which begins as a deep fissure or ulcer in Crohn's disease and progresses through the entire thickness of the bowel wall. If the inflammation is contained within the bowel wall and adjacent mesentery or extends locally into the abdominal cavity, an abscess is formed, which consists of bacteria, fecal contents from the intestinal lumen, and pus. The latter is formed in the reaction of surrounding tissue accumulating white blood cells. Abnormal communications, fistulas, may develop from the abscess cavity to another loop of intestine, to the skin, to another abdominal organ such as the kidney, ureter, urinary bladder or a genital organ such as the vagina or, more rarely, the uterus (Fig. 8).

The symptoms of an abscess or fistula depend on its location. An abscess usually produces fever, abdominal pain, and localized

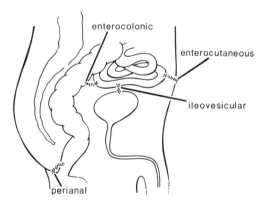

FIG. 8. Examples of Crohn's disease fistulas.

swelling (mass). The fever may be intermittent with high elevations and will often be accompanied by shaking chills or profuse sweating. Night sweats in which an individual perspires through his or her bed clothes and soaks the linens are typical manifestations of an abscess and represent nocturnal fevers. An abscess may remain hidden or produce an area of swelling and tenderness within the abdomen. Typically, the pus "looks for" an exit from the body and may "point," usually toward the abdominal wall. This will produce an area of swelling along the abdominal wall, which may become red, hot, and tender. Eventually, the abscess may drain spontaneously through the abdominal wall and, interestingly, may drain preferentially through a previous surgical incision (such as an appendectomy scar).

Common sites for abscesses in Crohn's disease are the perianal area and buttocks. In these locations, the abscess is painful, hot, and swollen. It makes the passage of a bowel movement uncomfortable, and an individual may have problems in sitting, walking, or finding any comfortable position. These abscesses occur because of burrowing inflammation from the rectum or anal canal and frequently recur after treatment.

The therapy for any abscess is surgical drainage. This may consist of a simple incision into the skin to allow the pus to drain or may require a more extensive operation depending on the location. A course of antibiotics is frequently prescribed, although antibiotics are rarely sufficient to heal a well-formed abscess without the accompanying drainage. Drainage alone may convert an abscess into a fistula, which may continue to leak or close spontaneously depending on the nature of the inflammation at the source within the bowel.

Fistulas may also occur without an abscess cavity when there is a direct extension of the ulcer through one loop of bowel to communicate directly with another loop of bowel, the skin, the genital area, or any of the structures mentioned above. Abscesses and fistulas occur in approximately one-fourth of patients with Crohn's disease and most commonly arise from the terminal ileum. The location of the ileum deep in the pelvis produces fistulas that communicate with the sigmoid colon, vagina, and, typically, the perianal area.

Fistulas may occur spontaneously in Crohn's disease and also are frequent after surgical procedures. Fistulas may occur in any area involved with Crohn's disease, and the symptoms and complications of such fistulas depend on their location. Fistulous communications between two loops of small intestine may produce no symptoms whatsoever. The physician may be able to feel thickened loops of bowel when examining the abdomen, and an X-ray study may demonstrate the abnormal tract. When fistulas occur between the small intestine and the colon, a short-circuiting of liquid intestinal content may occur, directing liquid bowel contents into the large bowel, where they mix with the solid or formed stool that is present. Such a patient would complain of a change in bowel habits with the drainage of liquid, often bile-stained stool along with formed stool or simply a worsening of diarrhea. The presence of bile is often irritating to the rectum and may cause burning in the anal area and surrounding skin.

A fistula to the urinary tract may produce symptoms similar to a urinary tract infection with fever, painful and frequent urination, and commonly, the passage of gas or stool along with urine. A fistula into the vagina will cause drainage of excess mucus, stool, or gas through the vaginal canal. In this location, fistulas may make sexual intercourse painful because of the adjacent inflammation.

When a fistula is about to exit through the skin, a local area of redness will develop with eventual skin breakdown. This may be followed by the drainage of intestinal contents or stool through the skin. The exact nature of the discharge will depend on how high within the intestinal tract the fistula originates. Often the drainage will be irritating to the skin and produce local pain and burning and additional skin breakdown.

Fistulas are diagnosed by a variety of methods. An X-ray examination of the intestine is obtained to define the underlying abnormalities of the bowel. The doctors may be able to identify the location of the fistula from routine X-ray studies alone. If this is not sufficient, additional studies (enteroclysis) may be necessary. For cutaneous (skin) fistulas, X-ray dye may be introduced directly into the skin opening and followed back to the portion of bowel from which it originates. For urinary tract fistulas, an intravenous pyelogram in which dye, administered through a vein, is concentrated and excreted through the kidneys will outline the kidneys, ureter, and bladder. Fistulous communications may be identified through their distortion of this system, or it may be necessary for a urologist (surgeon specializing in diseases of the urinary tract) to examine the bladder by introducing a scope through the urethra. He may then identify where the opening occurs within the bladder.

Fistulas into the vagina can be visualized by an examination of the female pelvis. If the opening is too small to be identified, other techniques such as the swallowing of blue dye may identify the opening after this dye eventually passes through the fistula into the vagina.

The treatment of most fistulas requires surgically removing the severely inflamed intestine from which the fistula arises. Frequently, the surgeon is able to reconnect the two adjacent pieces of intestine, although a temporary stoma (opening of the bowel to the abdominal wall) is sometimes required. In a few situations, fistulas are able to heal with a combination of medical therapy and bowel rest. The rationale is to minimize the intestinal contents, thus reducing the pressure and flow through the fistula. This may allow the fistula tract to close down gradually (collapse) and heal, and in rare situations it may heal completely. Unfortunately, we are not as successful in the medical treatment of the fistula as would be hoped, so that surgical therapy is frequently necessary.

Crohn's disease of the perianal area (fistulas, fissures, and hemorrhoids) is one of the more frustrating and embarrassing complications of the illness. Destruction of the anal sphincter by either burrowing infection or surgical drainage can cause incontinence with leakage of mucus, pus, or stool, which may interfere with social activities or intimate relationships. Some patients are required to wear absorbent pads or, in rare cases, diapers to accommodate the soilage. The initial treatment is usually conservative. Antibiotics are helpful to prevent extension of infection with localized abscesses, and sitz baths cleanse and soothe the anal area. Spontaneous drainage of these abscesses or fistulas is desired, although surgical drainage may be required for deeper infections. Bowel rest and hyperalimentation may be of great help in controlling the symptoms of severe perianal disease but are rarely curative. Extensive surgery or even colostomy is, at times, required to control the destructive process.

NONINTESTINAL COMPLICATIONS

Many of the extraintestinal complications of Crohn's disease are similar to those of ulcerative colitis and are reviewed again briefly. However, Crohn's disease involving the small intestine expands the spectrum of associated problems.

Minor liver disorders are frequent in Crohn's disease. Common abnormalities include mild inflammation within the small bile duct of the liver, termed pericholangitis, usually without symptoms; this may only be identified by the physician when performing routine liver blood tests. This abnormality is not known to progress to a more severe form of liver disease and usually will not influence the course of inflammatory bowel disease. Another form of mild liver disease is produced by fat infiltration into the liver, which occurs in extremely ill patients or those with poor nutritional intake over long periods of time. A "fatty liver" may evolve in patients who are receiving corticosteroids and is also a benign, asymptomatic, and totally reversible form of liver disease. Viral hepatitis may interrupt the course of Crohn's disease and is related to the number of blood transfusions. The great majority of individuals who develop hepatitis can be expected to recover without any ill effects, although a few patients may develop a chronic form of hepatitis that on occasion progresses to liver scarring or cirrhosis. The latter refers to a shrunken, irreversibly damaged liver that, to a variable degree, is unable to function fully. Sclerosing cholangitis is another more severe bile duct damage related to inflammation that involves the larger routes of drainage from the liver; it occurs rarely in Crohn's disease but does tend to progress to cirrhosis over long intervals of time (perhaps 10 to 20 years).

Arthritis in Crohn's disease is similar to that in ulcerative colitis and usually produces swelling and pain in larger joints such as the knees, hips, elbows, and wrists. Rarely does the arthritis produce lasting symptoms or joint destruction, and symptoms may coincide with flare-ups of the bowel condition. Sacroiliitis, an inflammatory

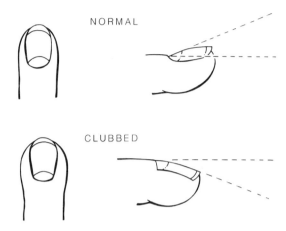

FIG. 9. Normal and clubbed fingernails.

arthritis of the lower back and spine, develops in fewer than 10% of patients with Crohn's disease. Again, it is related to a genetic marker (HLA-B27) and may cause low back pain associated with stiffness of the lower spine. It should be treated with a combination of antiinflammatory medications and a regular exercise program.

A very mild and painless swelling of the finger and toenails producing a peculiar spoon shape of the nail ("clubbing"; Fig. 9) may be associated with active bowel inflammation and will often resolve as the bowel disease is treated. Other changes in the nails, such as brittle, cracked, or creased nails, may be related to nutritional inadequacies.

Gallstones in the presence of Crohn's disease are related to the malabsorption of bile acids from the terminal ileum. This results in an increase in the concentration of cholesterol in the bile, which allows gallstones to crystallize in the gallbladder. These are usually without symptoms but may produce typical gallbladder attacks. When these occur, they must be differentiated from other symptoms of Crohn's disease and can be treated successfully by surgical removal of the gallbladder or, on occasion, by extraction of the stone through an endoscope.

Skin rashes occur with Crohn's disease as in ulcerative colitis. Erythema nodosum affects women more often than men, producing red or reddish-blue raised, warm, and tender nodules that are located more commonly on the lower legs, especially along the shins, and often in relation to local injury. These nodules, which often herald active bowel disease, may resolve spontaneously without treatment, although steroid injections or topical steroids will usually be necessary.

More severe ulcerating skin lesions called pyoderma gangrenosum affect the legs but may occur elsewhere. They are deep, painful, ulcerating areas of skin breakdown with an elevated purplish margin. These require intensive local treatment with frequent cleansing and topical antibiotics and steroids under the guidance of a skin specialist (dermatologist).

Many other nonspecific skin rashes may occur in the setting of Crohn's disease, such as eczema and hives. Psoriasis is not uncommon and may occur in other family members. They are at times bothersome but rarely of crucial significance and may reflect activity of bowel disease.

Small solitary or multiple ulcerations in the mouth similar to cold sores are called aphthous ulcers. Usually they produce only mild discomfort but can be painful and interfere with eating and drinking. Again, these usually occur with active bowel disease and may be associated with other skin rashes or eye problems. The latter include inflammation of the blood vessels of the eye (conjunctivitis), pupil (iritis), and sclera, the white portion of the eye (episcleritis). These eye problems usually respond to treatment with oral or topical steroids but require therapy by an experienced physician.

Problems with the kidney and genital organs occur more frequently in patients with Crohn's disease than in ulcerative colitis. Kidney stones develop in Crohn's disease when the terminal ileum is inflamed or removed surgically. These situations lead to malabsorption of fats, which then bind to calcium in the bowel. Under normal circumstances, free calcium in the bowel binds to dietary oxalate, preventing absorption, and the calcium–oxalate complex is then excreted in the feces. When the calcium is bound to fats, the free oxalate may be absorbed into the body and is then excreted through the kidneys. Within the kidneys the oxalate is concentrated and forms crystals, which may grow into stones within the urinary system. Manifestations of kidney stones are similar to those in noninflammatory-bowel-disease patients and usually presents as severe, crampy low back pain frequently associated with some blood in the urine. Kidney stones in these patients may be prevented by limiting the amount of fat and oxalate in the diet. Oxalate is present in spinach, tea, berries, and certain other leafy vegetables. Additional calcium supplementation may be helpful.

The urinary tract obstructions in Crohn's disease may be caused by an inflamed/swollen loop of bowel that compresses the right ureter draining the kidney. This usually will not induce symptoms and may be identified by special X-rays (intravenous pyelogram, IVP) or ultrasound examination of the kidneys. These investigations are important in certain individuals with Crohn's disease since the function of a kidney may be lost if obstruction persists over a long period of time. The obstruction may be treated by removal of the involved segments of bowel at surgery and is an indication for an operation in Crohn's disease.

Fistulas may occur too into the bladder in Crohn's disease, which may be suspected if patients pass blood, gas, or at times feces through the urine. Early symptoms include pain or difficulty in urination and must be differentiated from simple urinary tract infections.

Fistulas may occur too into the female genital tract in Crohn's disease, usually involving the vagina. As mentioned above, women may notice a discharge of additional mucus, gas, or at times, feces. In this situation, the symptoms are more troublesome than severe but should be evaluated.

Many of the symptoms of Crohn's disease are attributed to malnutrition. Weight loss, of course, is a sign of poor nutrition but is not necessarily present even when severe signs of individual nutrient loss occur. Typically, the terminal ileum is inflamed in Crohn's disease, causing poor absorption of vitamin B_{12} and eventually anemia. Vitamin D deficiency will cause osteomalacia (a weakening of the bones) that may be associated with bone pain, although this is often without symptoms in the early phases. Deficiencies in vitamin A produce difficulties in night vision, since this vitamin is important for the formation of cells that are involved with the reception of light within the retina of the eye. These symptoms are reversible with replacement of the vitamin. Malabsorption of vitamin K will produce bleeding problems, with easy bruising or bleeding of the gums as the first symptoms. Vitamin E deficiency is extremely rare but may cause a degeneration of nerves. All of these manifestations are treatable with supplements of vitamins and should be prevented by an adequate assessment of the diet and nutritional status of the patient at the time that Crohn's disease is first diagnosed by the physician.

Iron deficiency also is very common in inflammatory bowel disease as a result of a combination of loss of blood from intestinal bleeding and poor absorption when the small intestine is inflamed. Iron deficiency produces anemia, which may be prevented or treated by replacement of iron in one of three forms: iron tablets taken by mouth, iron given as a series of intramuscular injections, or intravenous infusions.

Zinc deficiency occurs in very severe Crohn's disease associated with significant malnutrition or with prominent fistula formation. Zinc deficiency may produce a variety of symptoms including alterations in taste sensation and hair growth, poor wound healing, or an unusual skin rash.

The more common effects of malnutrition are weight loss and muscle wasting. These frequently accompany abdominal pain and diarrhea. However, they may be a subtle manifestation of a poor appetite and a decreased intake to avoid symptoms. In children, growth may be delayed or retarded, and growth spurts may be stimulated by increasing the daily calorie intake.

Psychological problems are not unexpected in patients with inflammatory bowel disease. It is easy to understand how an individual with chronic or recurrent abdominal pain, diarrhea, rectal bleeding, or malnourishment would be depressed or overwhelmed by the uncertainties imposed by his or her disease. Emotional problems are often exacerbated by therapy with high doses of corticosteroids, which produce exaggerated mood swings, euphoria, or depression. Additionally, the threats of impending abdominal surgery or the necessity of a stoma are often overwhelming.

It does not appear, as was once taught, that a particular personality type or neurotic tendency will predispose an individual to

develop Crohn's disease. Nor does it seem that particular family
factors (e.g., a domineering mother or obvious family conflicts)
working on a vulnerable member are sufficient to induce bowel
inflammation. Rather, knowledge of early symptoms may be withheld because of fear or embarrassment, which may isolate the individual and be interpreted as a primary trait rather than a symptom
of the new disease. These problems will be discussed further (see
Chapter 11), and it should be clear that a supportive family environment is essential and that intermittent counseling of patients and
their families is often beneficial.

TREATMENT

The therapy of Crohn's disease must be viewed from both a short-
and long-term perspective. In the simplest sense, medical treatment
can be seen as an attempt to control the symptoms of Crohn's
disease, whereas surgery is utilized to treat many of the complications of the Crohn's disease inflammatory process (see Chapters 8 and 10).

The interaction and cooperation between the patient, family, gastroenterologist, and surgeon are even more important with Crohn's
disease than with ulcerative colitis. This arises from the fact that
Crohn's disease is not curable by either medical or surgical therapy
(e.g., compared to ulcerative colitis which is cured by colectomy)
and once surgery has been required, there is a significant risk of the
need for further operations.

The medical therapy for Crohn's disease is approached in the
same stepwise fashion as for ulcerative colitis. Diet can be considered the first line of defense, and a consistent diet that will help to
control each individual's symptoms will be very useful in reducing
the need for supplemental medications (most notably antidiarrheal
preparations). The exact dietary requirements and alterations are
discussed more fully in Chapter 9.

Many medications are available to assist in the control of symptoms in Crohn's disease. The most commonly prescribed are the
antispasmodic/sedative combinations such as phenobarbital and belladonna, Donnatal®, Bentyl®, Librax®, Combid®, among others.
These drugs help to reduce the abdominal pain, cramps, distention,

and occasional nausea. When patients are symptomatic, we believe that these medications should be utilized on a regular basis rather than taken intermittently "as needed." The regular schedule allows the maintenance of tissue levels to control the symptoms continually, whereas, patients taking the medications irregularly will notice that it may take longer for the medications to work or allow swings in the symptoms to occur (e.g., alternate days of diarrhea and constipation).

The antidiarrheal preparations, diphenoxylate (Lomotil®) and loperamide (Imodium®), are often used to control the frequency of bowel movements. The more potent opiate derivatives (deodorized tincture of opium, paregoric) and codeine preparations are sometimes required for more severe diarrhea, especially after major intestinal resections by surgery. The latter medications require a greater degree of control by the physician because of their potential for physical tolerance and addiction. This potential arises from their absorption into the body and the influence on opiate (pain) receptors in the brain. Furthermore, these medications have a potent effect on the intestinal tract and can act to increase the pressures within the bowel, actually intensify cramping, distention, and abdominal pain; most commonly in the setting of partial blockage of the bowel.

Medications for pain are, at times, necessary in Crohn's disease. Unfortunately, it is far easier to prescribe these medications than it is to control the underlying disease process. This frequently leads to longer term problems of pain control versus narcotic abuse in patients with longstanding Crohn's disease. We believe that potent narcotic pain medications should be avoided in the great majority of patients with Crohn's disease, except in the setting of pre- or postoperative care. We greatly prefer to treat the underlying condition producing the pain rather than masking the pain with medications which, in and of themselves, create additional problems.

Sulfasalazine (Azulfidine®) is a common, first line medication used to control the inflammation in Crohn's disease. As with ulcerative colitis, sulfasalazine appears to be more effective when the colon is involved although many of us have also found it to be useful when the small intestine is inflamed. The exact mechanism by which sulfasalazine is effective has yet to be totally clarified, although it does appear that the 5-aminosalicylic acid (5-ASA) component is able to reduce the chemical mediators of inflammation. Since the splitting of sulfasalazine into its two components (5-ASA and sulfapyridine) requires the presence of bacteria, either the transport of the drug into the colon or the presence of bacterial overgrowth in the small intestine (as commonly occurs in Crohn's disease) are needed to activate the drug.

Other anti-bacterial (antibiotic) medications are frequently used as adjuncts in the treatment of Crohn's disease. Although none of these medications have demonstrated a consistent antiinflammatory effect, the rationale for their use is to reduce the population of bacteria within the lumen of the bowel that could potentially gain entry into the inflamed bowel wall. Although many different antibiotics have been used empirically (tetracycline, ampicillin, Keflex®, Bactrim™, or Septra®) only metronidazole (Flagyl®) has been compared to sulfasalazine in a large clinical trial. Although Flagyl® has been touted for the use in perianal Crohn's disease, the drug has shown to be as effective as Azulfidine® for the primary treatment of Crohn's disease of the colon and small intestine in a Scandinavian study. Further evaluation of this medication as a primary treatment in Crohn's disease is currently being studied in the United States.

Corticosteroids remain the most effective medical therapy for Crohn's disease at present. These medications have been found to be useful in treating most aspects of active Crohn's disease by directly reducing the inflammatory response. This can result in a reduction of the degree of narrowing of the bowel and, hence, improving the cramps; with more pronounced mucosal inflammation, corticosteroids can "plug the mucosal leaks" and reduce the amount of diarrhea. Unfortunately, these medications provide their beneficial effects at the expense of a multitude of side effects as discussed elsewhere. It should be mentioned that corticosteroids have been shown to be effective only for the active phase of Crohn's disease and are not effective in either preventing recurrences of Crohn's disease once the inflammation has been controlled, nor are steroids indicated for the prevention of recurrences after surgical procedures when the active disease has been removed.

Immunosuppressive drugs (Imuran® and 6-mercaptopurine) have been used in Crohn's disease with a better outcome than in ulcerative colitis. We generally reserve these drugs for patients with longstanding or complicated Crohn's disease who have not responded adequately to the abovementioned medications. These drugs also have a role in a group of patients with Crohn's disease who are unable to wean off the steroids or who do not respond adequately to the introduction of steroids. Unfortunately, these medications are not as immediately effective as steroids are and may require up to six months for their full benefit to be evident. Furthermore, as our experience with these drugs increases, it seems as though many patients will "flare-up" as the drugs are withdrawn. Several groups, on the other hand, have been utilizing these agents earlier in the course of Crohn's disease with a fair degree of success. Their ultimate role in the treatment of Crohn's disease remains to be fully elucidated.

One form of nutritional therapy, hyperalimentation, also has been used in Crohn's disease and with more success than in ulcerative colitis. We have found hyperalimentation to be useful not only for patients with malnutrition; but for patients with hard to control Crohn's disease, with patients whose Crohn's disease has progressed despite a multitude of medications, and to prepare patients for anticipated surgical procedures. Many patients have obtained a long period of remission from their Crohn's disease after a course of total parenteral nutrition (TPN) and studies are currently underway to assess their optimal use in Crohn's disease.

SURGICAL THERAPY

The aim of surgical treatment in Crohn's disease is to deal with the complications of the illness that are not amenable to medical therapy. Although it was once felt that removal of the inflamed intestine may "cure" the underlying condition as occurs with ulcerative colitis, it is now realized that this is not the case. One can understand why surgery is not curative when it is understood that microscopic changes of Crohn's disease are apparent throughout the gastrointestinal tract in many patients with Crohn's disease and that only the most obvious site of active disease is removed at surgery. After a segment of intestine is removed (resected) and the adjoining loops of bowel are connected (anastomosed), there is a tendency for the inflammation to recur near the site of connection (anastomosis). The likelihood of the recurrence in Crohn's disease depends on how closely one observes the patient for subsquent inflammation. For instance, if one considers the risk of recurrence to be that of reoperation, this risk will be much less than if one observes the patient for the recurrence of X-ray, endoscopic, or even microscopic lesions. The actual risk of recurrence is difficult to state for an individual patient and relates to the age at which the first operation is performed, the length of time the patient has had Crohn's disease, the location of Crohn's disease (small bowel alone versus colon alone versus small intestine and colon), and the type of surgery performed (resection with anastomosis versus ileostomy).

Because of the reasons mentioned above surgery is generally indicated to treat the complications of Crohn's disease rather than as a primary mode of therapy. Such complications include a blockage of the bowel (obstruction), persistent bleeding, fistulas into adjoining structures (small intestine into colon, into the bladder or urinary tract, to the skin, or a severe fistula to the vagina, or severe disease around the anus), for growth retardation in children that does not respond to medical treatment, and in other cases where medical therapy fails.

In all cases, the optimal surgery is that which removes the least amount of bowel in order to preserve the remaining intestine. This rule is, again, in contrast to ulcerative colitis for which the entire colon is removed. In Crohn's disease, it is possible to remove only the inflamed segment and to reconnect the adjacent, healthy appearing bowel. At times, the entire colon may have to be removed, in which case an ileostomy may be performed. Again, unlike the situation with ulcerative colitis, if the rectum is spared in Crohn's disease, it is possible to connect the small intestine to the rectum (ileorectal anastomosis). On the other hand, anal sparing procedures and internal pouches are not possible in Crohn's disease due to the potential for inflammation to recur and invade these new structures.

After a surgical procedure in Crohn's disease, the patient usually returns to the care of his or her internist/gastroenterologist. Most patients, after having the inflamed segment removed, will again feel well and not require continued medical therapy after the pre-operative steroid dose has been completely tapered. Along these lines, no specific medications have been shown to be effective in preventing the recurrence of the inflammation in Crohn's disease. We, therefore, recommend continued good-health habits after surgery, including an emphasis on an adequate recuperative period, appropriate nutritional guidelines depending on the exact nature of the surgery (see Chapters 9 and 10) and continued follow-up with the physician. Often such procedures provide the patient a period of excellent health and renewed optimism after the stormy course that led to the operation.

PROGNOSIS

The outlook for an individual patient with Crohn's disease is variable. The future depends upon a number of factors including the age at which one develops symptoms of Crohn's disease, the location and extent of inflammation, complications arising during the course of Crohn's disease, and the individual's response to treatment. We see many individuals for whom Crohn's disease is a minor annoyance. They may have intermittent symptoms of abdominal cramps and need to watch their diet for foods that may aggravate their abdominal discomfort. On the other hand, some patients require constant treatment with high doses of steroids and other medications in order to control constant diarrhea. Others may require numerous operations to control frequent obstructions. And still other patients will have a single operation for "ileitis" and never have another problem again.

Most patients are somewhere in the middle with the need to watch their diet, to maintain good-health habits, and to take occasional medications. We always maintain an optimistic outlook and prefer to treat patients with early symptoms rather than to wait until the inflammatory process is so out of control that intensive medical (or surgical) therapies are needed.

Since many patients who develop Crohn's disease are young at the onset of their illness, the illness often comes at a critical time during a person's emotional development. Although most patients are able to "cope" to an almost unbelievable degree, at times additional support from a psychiatric nurse, social worker, or therapist will be needed to assure that personality development advances smoothly. An understanding and sympathetic family (spouse, parent, or sibling) are of great benefit. Some of these aspects are discussed more completely in Chapter 11.

Many young patients with Crohn's disease are concerned about the ability to have a family. Young men with Crohn's disease are usually normally fertile, although in rare instances medication taken for Crohn's disease may temporarily reduce the sperm count. Women with Crohn's disease can bear children without complication. There is little influence of the Crohn's disease on pregnancy, as long as the pregnancy is undertaken during a time of good health. The common medications used to control the symptoms of Crohn's disease (sulfasalazine and steroids) have been shown to be harmless to both the mother and the baby. The main consideration is to keep the mother in the best physical shape during pregnancy to assure a healthy infant. This includes good nutrition and weight gain for the mother and will often require close cooperation between the obstetrician and the gastroenterologist. It is only when women with active Crohn's disease conceive that the risk of early miscarriage is increased. There is no increased risk of birth defects due to the Crohn's disease or the usual medications used to control Crohn's disease, although all drugs need to be assessed on their individual merits compared to their potential consequences.

Many patients will be concerned about the chance of "passing" Crohn's disease onto their children. Although there is an increased prevalence of Crohn's disease within families in which one member has Crohn's disease there appears to be no specific chance of transmitting Crohn's disease from one family member to another. We do not believe that the slight possibility of a child developing inflammatory bowel disease is a sufficient reason to avoid having children if a couple so desires.

Most of our patients will persevere through some degree of adversity with their Crohn's disease, but most rise above the problem. We are always impressed with the "intestinal" fortitude of our patients who are capable of pursuing totally normal lifestyles, families, and jobs, despite their physical problems. In fact, one of the most inspiring aspects of caring for patients with Crohn's disease is to see the individual growth and willingness to provide mutual support with other patients. In this regard, the prognosis for Crohn's disease is excellent.

ADDENDUM

Crohn's Disease: A Patient's Perspective

Amy Amdur

Like most other eighteen-year-olds, my health was something I took largely for granted. In college, I was busy dividing my allotted twenty-four hours a day between university classes and my extra-curricular dance career. Life was fine.

Periodic abdominal pain then began to manifest itself in my life. At first, the pain seemed to coincide with due dates of papers, mid-terms and finals. Demanding high academic performance from myself, I did not allow the pain to interfere with my school work. I often waited until the middle of the night for the pain to end, so that I could begin to study. Relatives with good intentions suggested that the pain was psychosomatic. I even considered the possibility that my mind was the cause of the pain until the day pain forced me to turn back from the 10-minute walk to class. I realized then that the pain was real and that something was wrong. I decided to see a doctor as soon as possible.

My doctor quickly admitted me to a suburban hospital for tests. I had been hospitalized once before for illness; an emergency appendectomy. I knew something about hospital routine: nurses came in periodically to take my temperature, pulse and blood pressure; doctors made early morning visits en masse; various hospital employees visited, requesting payment for the television, insurance information, menu cards; blood work and urinalysis were done. I underwent my first humbling upper G.I. and lower G.I. X-ray series. The doctor diagnosed Crohn's disease.

I began asking questions: "What is Crohn's disease?" The answer: "A chronic and progressive inflammation of the G.I. tract." "What causes it?" The doctor shrugged his shoulders and said, "We don't know." "What is the cure?", I asked optimistically. Again, the response "We don't know." In my mind I asked, "Why me?" "What is the treatment?" At last, an answer: "The treatment is to control and contain the disease process.'' I learned that pharmaceuticals may be prescribed and may be effective in this regard. I began taking Azulfidine® and didn't notice any significant changes, except that my urine was orange.

Investigation and research into doctors and hospitals involved with Crohn's disease indicated that there was a doctor at the University of Chicago who was a specialist in Crohn's disease. I made an appointment and saw Dr. Kirsner. He wanted me to come to the hospital as an inpatient for tests. I was admitted and again underwent the upper and lower G.I. X-ray tests. I gave my medical history to one medical student after another. While hospitalized, I met other people with Crohn's disease. It was reassuring to talk with them. I found out that many of the things I had thought and experienced were commonalities between us. I wasn't so strange after all.

Dr. Kirsner concurred with the original diagnosis of Crohn's disease. He gave me a thorough explanation of Crohn's disease, what is known about the possible causes, the nature of the disease, different methods of treatment and long-term expectations. I learned that the nature of Crohn's was a chronic disease composed of periods of activity known as ''flare-ups'' and inactivity of little or no symptoms. I also learned that Crohn's is rarely fatal and that most people lead relatively normal lives. I had previously assumed that a progressive disease with no cure necessarily resulted in a shortened life. I was relieved to some degree.

Dr. Kirsner recommended that I take steroids to control the disease process. I asked about the side effects of steroids. I was told that while steroids are very helpful drugs in that they can control inflammation, they may have side effects that vary according to the individual. There is a tendency for a person on steroids to retain fluids. This creates the moon-face commonly seen on people who take this drug. Dr. Kirsner reminded me that the priority was to control the inflammatory process. I began taking steroids and took my medication exactly as prescribed. I immediately began to feel better; my appetite was insatiable. From time to time I experienced mood swings, a side effect of my medication. A fellow Crohn's patient had told me that she found it helpful to say mentally, ''It's the steroids'' whenever she experienced a particular ''high'' or ''low.'' She said that at first she had felt that she was going crazy when her mood would change from happy to sad without apparent cause. I found the mental reminder helpful.

Dr. Kirsner recommended that I follow a low-fiber, low-salt, low-residue, lactose-free, bland diet. Before leaving the hospital, I met with a hospital nutritionist. I wanted to find out specifically what I should and should not eat. Adherring to the highly restricted diet was much easier to do once the whys and wherefores had been explained to me.

I returned to college and led as normal a life as possible. I went to my classes. I drank water, instead of beer, at fraternity parties. When I felt good, I supplemented my academic classes with dance classes, rehearsals, and performances. When my health declined, I took life easier and adjusted my diet. When I had a flare-up, I restricted my activity and diet. I became one of the world's leading authorities on clear liquids, jello, magazines, and television.

My flare-ups were of varying degrees. Dr. Kirsner advised clear liquids and rest for the bad ones. I responded well to rest, warm weather and sunshine. I withdrew from college twice due to my inconsistent health status. I found it increasingly difficult to think about my future. There were times when, despite the fact that I took life easy, ate carefully, and took my medicine, I had flare-ups. Dr. Kirsner told me that I must remember that Crohn's disease is an aggressive disease. My flare-ups lasted 2–3 weeks. I perceived them as major interruptions in my life. They seemed to me to be roadblocks to my future.

I found myself experiencing depression more and more frequently. I was depressed because I had to deal with having a chronic illness. I was depressed by the recurring bouts of pain. When I was very sick, I wondered if I would ever get better. I was depressed that my life didn't seem normal anymore. My diet and activity were not what they had previously been. It was difficult for me to talk with my family and friends about these issues. I decided to see a therapist. During our sessions, I spoke about my fears and concerns related to Crohn's disease. My anxiety level was greatly reduced after talking about my feelings.

Dr. Kirsner suggested the possibility of surgery whenever I had a particularly bad flare-up. I was very afraid of surgery and worked hard to avoid it. I took the best care of myself possible. I ate well, slept well, took medicine, exercised, and maintained a positive attitude.

In spite of having Crohn's disease, I had many accomplishments during this time. I graduated from college. I choreographed, performed, swam, bicycled, maintained my own apartment, kept a busy social life. I began working, establishing what I hoped to be a normal life. I hoped that away from the pressures of college, my health would be under control. I continued seeing the doctor on a regular basis. My health vacillated between good and bad.

I began to become dissatisfied with the overall course of things. There was always a noticeable mass in the lower right quadrant of my abdomen that the doctors were concerned about.

Five years after my initial hospitalization, Dr. Kirsner suggested I return to the hospital for tests to review the Crohn's situation. I was quite against the idea of going into the hospital. I was depressed and afraid throughout the three weeks preceding my admission date. I had fears concerning the tests that would be done. Each test seemed to contain the word ''scope'' and consist of a tube being inserted into a body orifice. I also had fears that Dr. Kirsner would recommend surgery. I was depressed because I felt I had failed in the quest for good health.

I was admitted to the hospital. Blood was drawn and an EKG was taken. Tests were done over the next week. Again, the lower G.I. was an unpleasant experience for me. I was thankful that the other tests were not called for.

The tests indicated fistulas i.e., channels that grow off the main intestinal segment, and a very inflamed area in the lower abdomen. Dr. Kirsner recommended a surgical resection: removal of the diseased bowel segment and reconnection of remaining healthy intestine. He told me that fistulas left alone could be very dangerous, as they can grow into other body organs. I agreed to the surgery.

Subsequently, Dr. Kirsner recommended TPN, total parenteral nutrition, to prepare for the surgery. TPN allows complete rest of the bowel while nourishment (calories, vitamins, minerals) is infused intravenously through a semi-permanent catheter that is surgically placed into a vein in the chest. After a few days, I became accustomed to the tube and the necessary procedures to hook up and disconnect from the pump that controlled the rate of infusion. I was connected to the machine for 11 hours every night. My fixation on food passed in time, although my hunger and desire to eat never diminished.

I used the time before surgery (three weeks) in a number of ways. To prepare my body, I went to physical therapy daily. My activities were planned and monitored by a physical therapist. I wanted to be in the best physical condition possible for the operation. I worked hard to maintain and build my strength through exercise. My personal theory was that the stronger I was when I went into surgery, the quicker I would bounce back post-operatively.

My mental attitude was positive. Through my doctor's arrangement, I met a woman about my age who had gone through the same procedure ten weeks earlier. She was doing well; she looked healthy and stated the same.

Seeing her and listening to her account of the operation was reassuring to me. It was one thing to speak to doctors who performed the surgery and another to speak to a person who had undergone the operation.

My surgery was scheduled first thing on a Monday morning. I was back in my room by early afternoon. In the late afternoon I got out of bed and walked down the hall. I got out of bed two more times that evening, walking further each time. I was determined to get better quickly. I knew that walking would expedite the removal of my N.G. (nasogastric) tube that had been inserted during surgery. The N.G. tube aspirated gastric juices post-operatively. The N.G. tube was more a nuisance than anything else.

Four days after surgery doctors determined that my bowels were working again and removed the N.G. tube. I continued to receive fluid through my TPN line. Five days after surgery, I began drinking small quantities of a high-nutrition drink. One week after surgery, I ate eggs and toast. The TPN line was removed, as I was able to receive nourishment by mouth. Remarkably, my body digested and processed the food normally. I was very happy! Nine days after surgery, I went home. I rested, went for walks, and ate good food. One month after surgery, I went swimming.

Over the past six years, I have learned many answers to my original question: "What can I do to help myself?" I found it very helpful to talk with other people who have Crohn's disease. Through this type of interaction, I learned that many of my thoughts and concerns were held by others. I met some of these people through N.F.I.C., the National Foundation of Ileitis and Colitis. N.F.I.C. is a voluntary, non-profit organization devoted to research into inflammatory bowel disease, and to the education of patients, physicians, and the public. There are 40 chapters nationwide. N.F.I.C. publishes informative pamphlets on different aspects of IBD.

Learning as much as possible about the nature of Crohn's disease and related topics permitted me to act as an informed, educated, active patient. I attended lectures on IBD. I read articles on IBD. I studied nutrition and better understood the rationale behind my restricted diet. I asked my doctors and pharmacist about the nature and function of my prescribed medications. I learned specific information pertaining to each drug, as well as the importance of timely and consistent administration of medications. I acted accordingly. Medication is helpful only when taken, and taken properly.

Through a close working relationship with my doctors, I felt involved and responsible in my health care. I did not expect the doctors alone to make me well. I believed that through a partnership between my doctors and myself, with each party taking an active role, I would receive the best care possible. I tried not to dwell on the question "Why me?" preferring to ask "What can I do for myself?"

Supportive family and friends are extemely helpful to a person with chronic illness. The nature of Crohn's and the repeated flare-ups over time is distressing to the afflicted individual. There may be occasions when a person with Crohn's becomes ill in a social or work setting. The individual must often change or cancel plans as health dictates. Chronic illness is experienced differently by individuals. Often, people feel a loss of control and a sense of helplessness when faced with continued periodic illness. Life is interrupted and plans are disturbed. Fears and depression are frequently seen as a result. In my case, I found it difficult to speak with family and friends about my health. As I mentioned earlier, I eventually saw a therapist. As my illness indirectly involved my family, I invited them to a few sessions.

The need for dependency versus independence is, at times, an issue in the course of a chronic illness. During bad times, the person with Crohn's is forced to give up a certain amount of control and be dependent on others for assistance. If hospitalized, control is limited even more. Hospital routine combined with the person's poor physical health result in limited decision-making ability on the patient's part. To counter these periods of dependence, I strive to be as independent as possible when able.

I believe it is important to take responsibility for yourself and take control of your life whenever possible. Times of poor health also prevent the individual's participation in exercise and sports. When health and doctors permit, I have found it extremely satisfying to follow a sensible exercise program. Dr. Kirsner recommended swimming, a good cardiovascular and respiratory workout. I have found swimming to be a very relaxing activity and good for managing stress. The chronically ill person may feel angry or ashamed of his or her body. Exercise seems to have a positive influence on a person's body perception.

Today, more and more people feel a need to take greater responsiblity for their health. It seems to me that it is especially important for the person with Crohn's to strive to be in the best health at all times. I have developed a special "10 Commandments" for the person with Crohn's disease.

1. Eat well. Follow your doctor's recommendations. Seek specific answers to questions you may have. Nutritionists and dieticians are excellent references.

2. Get enough sleep. We all need time for our bodies to rest.

3. Relax. Stress is unavoidable in our modern-day world. Take extra care to balance stress with relaxation.

4. Exercise as allowed. Exercise benefits both mind and body.

5. Socialize as able. Friends and normal activities help one's mental attitude. See yourself in the non-patient role when possible.

6. Get thoughts out. Talk or write about your feelings. Don't be a pressure-cooker. Anxiety is often reduced when the causing thought is shared.

7. See your doctor as scheduled. Avoiding your doctor or denying your illness will not necessarily "make it go away."

8. Take medications as prescribed. Although your doctor may prescribe a medicine, it will only work if you take it and take it correctly.

9. Be honest with your doctor. Your doctor relies on your own health report. When treating you, your report will keep your doctor abreast of your health and any changes.

10. Be an active participant in your health care. Don't expect your doctor to make everything better. Act as partners in your health care.

As a person living with the realities of chronic illness, I have learned the importance of the quality of one's life. Flare-ups are unpredictable and cannot be completely avoided. The time one has when feeling good is precious. The quality of my life between flare-ups is under my control. I strive to do as much as I can, to live life to the fullest when my health permits. I do not dwell on the bad times. Instead, I focus on the good times! I am optimistic about my future. I try to have as normal a life as possible. I no longer take my health or my life for granted. I see life as a gift to be enjoyed.

CHAPTER 8

Medical Therapy

Our concept of treatment of inflammatory bowel disease is based on a comprehensive program rather than exclusive dependence on drugs. A stepwise approach to the medical treatment of inflammatory bowel disease is aimed at reducing or avoiding the usage of the more potent medications in order to prevent potential side effects. Many measures are available to reduce the *symptoms* of inflammatory bowel disease without necessarily altering the inflammatory reaction itself. These approaches help the individual feel better while reducing the stress involved with the illness and therefore assist in the overall healing process. Most of these measures are directed at reducing the abdominal pain and diarrhea of both ulcerative colitis and Crohn's disease and should be used in conjunction with the dietary recommendations described in Chapter 9.

NONSPECIFIC FACTORS

We frequently prescribe mild anticholinergic medications for the relief of abdominal cramping and diarrhea. These drugs reduce the amount of muscle spasm within the bowel. There are numerous products along these lines (e.g, Donnatal®, Bentyl®, Pro-Banthine®, Combid®). Tincture of belladonna is liquid and is prescribed in a "dropper" form to allow an adjustable dose for each individual. Since most patients are quite sensitive to these products, we prefer such flexibility, although there are so many products now on the market that it is often easy to find an alternative medication for specific patients. Often these drugs are combined in pill form with a mild sedative such as phenobarbital or one of its derivatives. We feel that these medicines work most effectively in concert to relieve both the abdominal cramping pain as well as the anxiety that the pain often provokes.

Common side effects of the anticholinergic (antispasmodic) drugs include a dry mouth because of decreased production of saliva and blurred vision. A rapid heart beat or palpitations may also occur in a few individuals receiving higher doses. Such drugs should be used cautiously in patients with glaucoma or certain forms of heart disease. When these drugs are used in conjunction with sedatives, drowsiness is an anticipated effect, which is more profound initially and usually improves after continued use.

These medications should be used with extreme caution in patients with severe or very active bowel disease. Likewise, in the presence of worsening symptoms, medications that inhibit the bowel function can induce a toxic dilatation (see Chapter 6) and should be used judiciously and only under the direct management of a physician.

Antidiarrheal medications such as diphenoxylate (Lomotil®) or loperamide (Imodium®) are commonly prescribed to reduce the number of loose or unformed bowel movements. These drugs function mainly by enhancing the absorption of water from the intestine, although there is some additional reduction of intestinal muscular activity. They are highly effective in reducing the number of bowel movements under most circumstances and can even cause constipation in patients with inflammatory bowel disease. They are potent drugs and should be taken under the direction of a physician; they may also cause dry mouth and/or blurred vision.

Psyllium (Metamucil® and other products) is a "bulk forming" compound produced from refined grain that retains water within the stool. The action can be helpful in preventing both diarrhea and constipation. Although it seems contradictory, both activities can be explained. By absorbing water like a sponge, bulk agents can soak up the free water within the intestinal lumen and hold the water within the compacted stool. This can be helpful in certain situations of watery diarrhea in both ulcerative colitis and Crohn's disease. On the other hand, in the patient with constipated bowel movements, the additional water retained within the stool helps to lubricate the fecal material, producing a softer and more easily eliminated bowel movement. The latter situation pertains especially to patients with proctitis, where the harder stools actually induce more bleeding. Here, these agents may be used on a trial basis beginning with small doses (e.g., 1 teaspoon). The dose may be adjusted upwards or downwards until the optimal effect is achieved. If symptoms worsen, the drug is stopped. These products should be avoided in patients with bowel narrowing, strictures, or possible obstruction, as the additional bulk within the intestine may produce a blockage.

Numerous stool softeners on the market (Colace® and others) act in a similar fashion, holding water within the stool. These may be helpful in certain situations, but patients must be careful to avoid products that have additional ingredients that may actually stimulate bowel activity. Such laxatives should be avoided in nearly all cases of inflammatory bowel disease.

In individuals in whom the terminal ileum has been removed, the loss of the last portion of the intestine as well as removal of the ileocecal valve may produce a more continuous flow of small intestinal contents into the colon. At the same time, bile salts, usually absorbed back into the system from the ileum, may pass into the large intestine. In the colon, the bile salts are converted to bile acids by colonic bacteria. Bile acids often are irritating to the colon and may produce increased secretion of fluid into the lumen and, hence, diarrhea. One means of preventing this is by the use of cholestryamine (Questran®). This medication is a resin that binds to bile salts and prevents their conversion to bile acids. Cholestyramine should be mixed completely in a liquid, and the exact dosage must be regulated individually in order for it to act most efficiently. Since the drug is a resin, it will also bind in a nonspecific manner to other drugs and fat-soluble vitamins. It should be used, again, under the direction of a physician and taken at times separate from taking other vitamins and medications so that their absorption will not be impaired. Cholestyramine also should be used with caution in patients with strictures or possible obstruction. As with any medication, the dosage scheduling is important to obtain the optimal results; therefore, the physician should be consulted regarding the appropriate timing related to meals and other drugs.

Pain relief is often a controversial issue in patients with inflammatory bowel disease, especially in Crohn's disease. A wide variety of pain medications are available to be utilized with the diet and other medications. A major concern, however, is the use of narcotics or other potentially addictive pain medicines. Since inflammatory bowel disease is a chronic problem, we unfortunately are confronted with patients who are referred to us who already are taking such medications and have become tolerant to the point that higher and higher doses are needed in order to be effective. Such potent medications have significant effects on bowel activity, which in many cases are counterproductive, such as spasm of the bowel muscles and increased pressure within the intestine produced by narcotics.

It is the intention of physician and patient alike to attain pain relief in patients with these uncomfortable illnesses. However, every attempt should be made to obtain the benefits of a specific diet program in conjunction with the agents described earlier prior to the administration of potentially addictive medications. There also is a strategy of using less potent analgesics such as acetaminophen[1] and other aspirin-like (but not aspirin–see later discussion) products and combination products, which are often quite beneficial. Beyond these, any pain medicines should be taken only under the direction of a physician. We should emphasize that severe, intractable (untreatable) pain be constantly reevaluated by the patient's doctor in order to explain the exact cause of the pain and permit consideration of potentially treatable causes that may have been overlooked. It is an extraordinarily rare patient who requires constant pain relief in any of these disorders, and such significant discomfort should make the patient and physician reconsider the option of surgery to avoid a long-standing requirement for narcotic medication.

It is also important for a patient with inflammatory bowel disease to avoid any medications (such as over-the-counter products) with-

---

[1]Tylenol®, Panadol®, Anacin 3®, Datril®, are examples.

out consulting his or her doctor. Many of these may have unanticipated harmful effects on the bowel. One such example is
aspirin,[2] which may cause ulcers in the esophagus, stomach, and
small bowel while, at the same time, impairing the blood-clotting
action of platelets and may induce or aggravate bleeding tendencies.
The doctor attending to the bowel disorder also should be made
aware of any medications prescribed by other physicians so that he
or she can anticipate any drug interactions or effects on the bowel.
For instance, certain antibiotics (such as penicillin) should be
avoided unless absolutely necessary, as they may cause diarrhea and
intensify or precipitate a flare-up of the underlying ileitis or colitis.

CORTICOSTEROIDS

Steroids are derivatives of the natural body hormone (chemical
messenger) cortisone, produced in the adrenal gland. The role of
this essential hormone is to facilitate the capacity of the metabolic
systems of the body to deal with stress. To do so, cortisone and its
related compounds must influence virtually all of the organ systems
of the body. These chemicals are constantly being produced by the
adrenal gland, though in varying amounts in a cyclical rhythm, so
that more hormone is produced in the early hours of the morning
with decreasing amounts through the day and the lowest level in the
evening and night. One of the effects of the cyclical production is
the wakefulness early in the day and fatigue by late afternoon or
evening.

There are many influences on this daily production of cortisone.
One example is stress, which may be in the form of either emotional
unrest or physical illness. In these situations, the body produces
more cortisone, which enhances the individual's defenses against
illness. Cortisone has a major influence on the liver and establishes
the chemical balance such that glucose (a primary food source for all
organs in the body) is liberated more freely. Cortisone also tones the
nervous system by enhancing the production of additional chemical

---

[2]Found in Bufferin®, Anacin®, Alka-Seltzer®, selected cold tablets, among
others.

messengers such as epinephrine (adrenalin), which can heighten an individual's reflexes but also produces a nervous or "hyper" sensation.

Abnormalities in the adrenal gland causing overproduction of cortisone have the same consequences as large doses of steroid medication. This condition, known as Cushing's disease, can produce an altered physique with a "moon face," additional body and facial hair, acne, purple-colored skin lines called stria, and altered fat distribution with fat along the back of the neck (termed a buffalo hump) as well as internal changes such as thinning of the bones, a tendency toward higher blood sugar (diabetes), and blood pressure elevation (hypertension).

The use of steroids for the treatment of inflammatory bowel disease stems from the fact that in high doses these chemicals have a potent antiinflammatory action. In a nonspecific manner, steroids inhibit the production of chemical mediators of inflammation, which interferes with the reactions of certain populations of white blood cells. This is the source of the major benefit of these drugs in inflammatory bowel disease, but also accounts for the increased susceptibility to infections when individuals are continuously taking higher doses.

Steroids are the most powerful medications in the physician's current armamentarium for inflammatory bowel disease. However, because of their numerous other influences on the body, they are also the most controversial. Steroids have a terrible reputation from the patient's standpoint because of these numerous other effects. Most individuals dislike the redistribution of fat and the facial hair and puffiness that accompany steroid usage as well as the exaggerated emotional trends that are often induced when large quantities of these drugs are prescribed. On the other hand, for patients who are quite ill, the introduction of steroids usually evokes a rapid therapeutic response, coinciding with the diminished inflammatory reaction, that includes an enhanced appetite, feeling of well-being, reduction of pain, and improvement in most symptoms.

Because of their potency, steroids must be used with caution and under the direction of a physician. Most commonly, these medications are given initially in higher doses (e.g., prednisone 40 to 60 mg/dosage) to provide a rapid and intense antiinflammatory response. As the disease is controlled, the medication is tapered to allow the body's own defenses to take over the healing process. Too rapid decrease of the medications will often produce flare-ups. Continuation of high doses produces side effects, which may not be tolerable in the long term. At each level the physician must weigh the potential benefit and the risk of this (and any) treatment and continue to consider other medical or surgical therapeutic options.

From the patient's point of view, once embarked on a treatment program involving steroids, the individual must be aware that he or she is on a potent medication that requires careful management. When one takes steroids in large doses, the natural production of cortisone by the adrenal gland is reduced. This change occurs over many days and weeks and will require a similar time period to recover. The sudden discontinuation of large doses of steroids does not allow the body sufficient time to recover its own production of cortisone. This leaves the individual in a very susceptible condition should any stress arise. Even a modest infection or injury, in the absence of cortisone, could produce shock. Rapid dehydration, low blood sugar, high fever, and abnormalities in the blood electrolytes (salts) could ensue and even lead to death. Part of the reason for the slow tapering of steroids is to allow the gradual production of cortisone in the adrenal gland to resume and increase and take over once the prescribed dose is below the level usually released by the adrenal gland.

Steroids may be administered in a variety of ways. When individuals are acutely ill or cannot take medications by mouth, cortisone[3] may be given intravenously or intramuscularly by injection. In an enema form, these drugs also have a topical action similar to cortisone cream applied to a skin rash. Hence, enemas are frequently given to patients with inflammation of the lower colon and rectum. Most commonly, however, the medications are given in a pill form. Various preparations of different potency and length of action are available. In some situations another hormone, ACTH,

---

[3]Hydrocortisone (Solu-Cortef®), prednisone (Deltasone®), methylprednisolone (Medrol®), etc.

may be given as injections, which stimulates tne adrenal gland's production of cortisone to similarly high levels. ACTH can only be given for short periods of time without inducing enlargement of the size of the adrenal gland while producing essentially the same results as prednisone (or other steroids) by mouth.

The potential undesirable effects of steroids are related to the dosage, length of time on the medication, as well as the individual's tolerance and response to the treatment. No two persons will react in the same manner to any particular dosage of these drugs, and the state of illness and nutritional status of the patient also will influence the response to these medications. Additionally, one must remember that some of the effects of these drugs, which are anticipated and felt to be beneficial by the physician (such as increased appetite and weight gain), may be interpreted as undesirable and unwanted by an individual patient.

The spectrum of side offects is wide, reflecting the action of steroids on all body tissues. Most patients will notice an increased appetite and rapid weight gain. A redistribution of body fat can produce facial puffiness, more fat in the midbody (chest, back, and abdomen), and relatively thin arms and legs. Increased facial hair may be most disturbing to women, and an enhanced disposition towards the development of acne (pimples) is equally disturbing to both sexes.

Aside from the abovementioned influence on a patient's appearance, there are numerous affects of steroids on the body's metabolism. Steroids cause retention of salt by the kidneys, which may lead to higher blood pressure. These medicines may also heighten (or unmask) the tendency towards high blood sugar levels (diabetes). The formation of cataracts is hastened, and there are several effects on the muscles and bones. Since cortisone is a catabolic (breakdown) steroid, compared, for example, to testosterone, the male anabolic (build-up) steroid, it is not possible to strengthen or add bulk to the muscles while on high doses. Likewise, there is a tendency for thinner bones because of the gradual loss of bone material. The latter may lead to more brittle, weaker bones, which can more easily be fractured or collapse.

The influence of steroids on the immune system also will impair some of the body's defense system against infections. This is seen only in very high doses of prednisone and may be most significant for patients whose resistance is already low. Conversely, it must be remembered that as the beneficial effects take over, all of the abovementioned "bad" effects are reversed, with the end result of a healthier, happier patient. This implies that these medications are to be used judiciously by experienced physicians who are able to regulate the dosages to the ultimate advantage of the patient and who can anticipate the potential consequences of these drugs and avert the most severe reactions in informed, cooperative patients.

ANTIBACTERIAL AGENTS

Sulfasalazine (Azulfidine®) is a combination of two different compounds linked together by a chemical bond. Although the drug is not a true antibacterial agent, it is included in this category because one of the components is a sulfa antibiotic (sulfapyridine). The other ingredient, 5-aminosalicylic acid (5-ASA), is a salicylate related to aspirin. When the parent compound is taken by mouth, the drug is only minimally absorbed from the small intestine. When sulfasalazine reaches the colon, however, the compound is split by colonic bacteria into the two separate chemical compounds. A majority of the sulfapyridine is then absorbed into the bloodstream and is eventually metabolized by the liver and excreted (eliminated) through the kidneys. The 5-ASA remains within the large bowel and appears to be the effective antiinflammatory agent.

Whereas the 5-ASA portion of sulfasalazine provides the therapeutic benefit, it is the sulfapyridine that accounts for the majority of the adverse effects accompanying this medication. Although most individuals tolerate sulfasalazine without significant side effects, many people develop headaches, nausea, or gastrointestinal upset. A few individuals have allergic reactions including skin rashes that are typical of sulfa allergies, hepatitis, or anemia, all of which are related to the sulfapyridine.

Sulfasalazine has been proven to be of benefit in the treatment of ulcerative colitis. This medication is helpful especially in mild or moderate ulcerative colitis. In very severe cases, the drug usually is withheld until the symptoms begin to improve. Sulfasalazine has been shown to be effective in bringing about remission in ulcerative colitis as well as in maintaining remission for up to several years after a flare-up. If the drug is stopped during the first year of illness, there is greater than a 50% likelihood that the colitis will reactivate.

Initially, sulfasalazine is given in a dosage of between 2 and 4 g (4 to 8 tablets) daily. After the symptoms have quieted down, the dosage may be reduced to 2 g (4 tablets) daily and should be continued for up to several years thereafter.

In Crohn's disease, sulfasalazine has been shown to be effective in the treatment of colitis as well as of small intestinal Crohn's disease when the ileum is involved, although less decisively than in ulcerative colitis. Sulfasalazine has been shown to be of benefit in the treatment of active Crohn's disease, although this medication is not of proven benefit in the prevention of exacerbations of inactive disease (remissions) or after surgery. Despite this lack of proven efficacy, many physicians will continue a patient on sulfasalazine even after the acute episodes have quieted down.

The common, nonallergic side effects (nausea, stomach upset, headache) can be minimized *when sulfasalazine is taken with a meal*. Because of a slight increased risk of kidney stones in patients taking sulfa medications (as well as the increased susceptibility to kidney stones in patients with inflammatory bowel disease), patients should drink a large amount of water or fluids throughout the day to maintain adequate hydration. The physician will also probably wish to perform a blood test several weeks after initiating therapy with sulfasalazine to make certain that the blood count is not affected by this medication.

Another possible undesirable affect of sulfasalazine in men is an abnormal sperm count. Alterations in both sperm appearance and motility have been identified in some individuals taking this drug. This probably accounts for some cases of infertility occurring while patients are on this medication, and these abnormalities are reversible and disappear after the drug is discontinued. There have been no instances of birth defects or spontaneous abortions (miscarriages) that are directly related to the medication, and many men have sired offspring and women have become pregnant and had completely normal pregnancies and deliveries. Hence, birth control should certainly be continued (if desired). Although no medication is desirable during pregnancy, the importance of maintaining adequate control over inflammatory bowel disease during a pregnancy outweighs the small risks of continuing the medication.

Some of the sperm abnormalities are to be related to another effect of sulfasalazine, the impairment of absorption of folic acid from the diet. Folic acid is an important vitamin for the production of red blood cells, nerves, and rapidly growing cells of the body such as the mucosal lining of the intestinal tract. Whenever a patient is placed on sulfasalazine, he should take an additional 1 or 2 mg daily of folic acid to compensate for the impaired absorption.

Aside from sulfasalazine, no other antibacterial medication is of proven benefit for ulcerative colitis. However, in patients who are allergic to sulfa or who cannot tolerate the drug, we will frequently use an alternative antibiotic based on the consideration that although bacteria are unlikely to be the cause of colitis, a reduction in the amount of bacteria may be helpful in healing the bowel. Alternatives include other sulfa preparations, tetracyclines (Achromycin®), erythromycin, or metronidazole (Flagyl®). In severe cases of toxic megacolon or colitis that require hospitalization, antibiotics are often given intravenously to enhance the benefit of corticosteroids and to prevent bloodstream infection.

In Crohn's disease we also use antibiotics as a component of medical therapy. In this setting, metronidazole has been shown, in European studies, to be as effective as sulfasalazine in the treatment of mild to moderate disease without the use of steroids. Metronidazole is an antibiotic that has been used for many years in the treatment of vaginal infections in women and is also very effective as an antibiotic against certain bacteria that do not require oxygen (anaerobes). Metronidazole may produce a metallic taste in the mouth and occasional nausea. An important side effect that requires a reduction in the dose or discontinuation of the drug is peripheral neuropathy (impairment of the nerve), which can cause a tingling or numbness of the fingers, hands, toes, or feet. Consumption of alcohol should be avoided while taking metronidazole because of a metabolic effect of this medication that can cause profound nausea and vomiting when taken with alcoholic compounds. Metronidazole has been shown to cause cancer and birth defects when given in large amounts in some laboratory animals. However, no such harmful effects have been documented in humans who have taken the drug safely over weeks and months. It is recommended that women taking this medication use some form of reliable contraception, and the drug should definitely be stopped if the woman is considering pregnancy or if she becomes pregnant while taking metronidazole.

Other antibiotics (e.g, tetracycline, ampicillin) also are frequently used as adjunctive treatment for Crohn's disease, although a proven benefit has yet to be shown. Again, they are used under the assumption that a reduction in the bacterial contents of the bowel will be helpful by reducing the inflammatory reaction and preventing contamination of the bloodstream with bacterial products. Future studies are needed to evaluate adequately the role of newer and more selective antibacterial products other than sulfasalazine and metronidazole for the treatment of inflammatory bowel disease.

IMMUMOSUPPRESSIVE AGENTS

Two drugs, azathioprine (Imuran®) and 6-mercaptopurine (6-MP, Purinethol®), are considered to be immunosuppressive drugs because of their ability to reduce or impair the function of a population of immune reactive cells in the body. These effects are more prominent in high doses, which are usually administered for the treatment of various forms of cancer. Over the past decade these drugs have also been used in much lower doses for the treatment of inflammatory bowel disease. Although a large, multi-center study of the effectiveness of Imuran® in Crohn's disease did not show any advantage of this drug when given over a short period of time, several groups of investigators working with inflammatory bowel disease have found these medications to be of benefit in the long-term treatment of complicated patients with Crohn's disease and ulcerative colitis. One of the major benefits has been to allow a reduction in the dose of steroids while taking Imuran® or 6-MP.

It appears that a certain proportion of patients who have not responded to other medications will improve with either of these drugs. However, it may take from six months to a year for the full benefit to be achieved. Additionally, many patients will "flare-up" as the medicines are tapered in dose, similar to the "flare-ups" after tapering prednisone.

These medications have been used quite successfully, without severe complications, in relatively low doses, with relatively few side effects. The concern over these medicines, however, is the potential for severe, albeit rare, side effects that have been recognized, as well as some potential long-term effects that have not been completely evaluated. In the initial multi-center study, Imuran® was taken off the protocol when a significant number of patients developed pancreatitis, an inflammation of the pancreas, which was unrelated to the Crohn's disease. Furthermore, in higher doses these medications lower all of the blood counts including the white blood cell and platelet counts. The latter reactions can make the patient susceptible to infections and to bleeding. Therefore, any patient taking these medicines requires continued monitoring of blood counts while on therapy.

The major long-term concern over these medicines is the possibility that they may alter the immune system's ability to defend against malignancies. This concern arises from the observation that patients with other diseases (e.g., kidney transplant patients) treated with immunosuppressive drugs are susceptible to the development of a variety of cancers. It should be noted that these patients are treated with many other medications as well, and may be susceptible to these problems unrelated to the immunosuppressive therapy. In any event, despite the concern, no malignancy has been directly linked to Imuran® or 6-MP therapy at the doses prescribed for inflammatory bowel disease. In addition, these medicines have definitely been linked to birth defects in animals who are taking the drugs and, therefore, these medicines should not be taken by men or women attempting to bear children while on the medication. Pregnancy should be delayed until a number of months after the drugs have been discontinued.

Despite these "potential" problems with these medications there does appear to be a role for immunosuppressive therapy in patients with complicated inflammatory bowel disease. We have seen some remarkable responses in individuals who have been able to fully taper steroids for the first time in their course of IBD and who have continued to do well for years. It is clear that medical investigators will continue to evaluate the appropriate setting, timing, dose, supplementary drugs, and consequences of this class of medications used for both Crohn's disease and ulcerative colitis.

CHAPTER 9

Diet and Nutrition

The role of nutrition and diet in inflammatory bowel disease is discussed frequently yet often misrepresented. There are no specific dietary factors that, as yet, have been definitely proven to cause or worsen either Crohn's disease or ulcerative colitis. On the other hand, adjustments of the diet help control such symptoms of inflammatory bowel diseases as abdominal cramps and diarrhea. Any such dietary alteration must take into account the potential nutritional deficiencies that occur secondary to bowel disease as well as the nutritional elements that may be omitted in restricted diets.

Before we proceed to a discussion of nutritional concepts related to inflammatory bowel disease, certain general considerations should be kept in mind. First, in normal individuals who consume a "well-balanced" diet, we are not aware of any specific nutritional deficiencies that arise. Any general diet will supply essential nutrients for individuals capable of digesting and absorbing normally. No specific supplementations (or vitamin preparations) have been found to be required for the maintenance of health or prevention of disease. It is only when individuals stray from a balanced diet and begin to avoid certain foods that potential deficiencies can occur. Even then, only a prolonged severely restricted diet may produce a specific deficiency in an otherwise normal individual (e.g., strict vegetarians who avoid all animal products only rarely develop vitamin B_{12} deficiency, and certain "formula" diets may not supply adequate amounts of essential minerals such as potassium. On the other hand, we have no problem in accepting daily use of a single multiple vitamin tablet since there are no side effects to a limited vitamin supplementation and the cost is quite low. Megavitamin preparations are of no proven value in maintaining health or preventing disease in the general population and can be potentially harmful.

Of course, patients with inflammatory bowel disease have increased need for nutritional supplementation because of the increased requirements imposed by illness and loss of essential nutrients through the inflamed bowel. It is for these individuals especially that the following discussion is directed with a reminder that the same basic principles apply to everyone.

The first principle dates to Einstein's observations about the conservation of mass. He recognized that all matter can be either converted into another form of mass or into energy. Likewise, energy can be derived from either a source of matter or another form of energy (e.g., coal into heat, electricity, then light; or sunlight into plant energy, which can be consumed by animals). During these transformations, the total amount of energy and matter remains constant. As related to these laws of nature, each person requires a certain amount of food to maintain his or her weight. If you do not eat anything, you will lose weight, whereas if you consume more food than you require to support your daily activity (energy), you will gain weight (mass).

Using the above principle, we are able to define an approximate requirement of food calories for each individual depending on his or her base-line or desired weight and activity schedule. For instance, larger individuals need more food to maintain their weight than smaller individuals, and people of the same size who have different activities will not require the same amount of calories (an athlete will require more food than a sedentary individual). It is also important to realize that during illness the body actually needs extra amounts of food to adjust to the increased metabolic demands of a fever, of "fighting off" an infection, or dealing with an inflammatory process. Hence, sick individuals will often need up to twice the number of calories as healthy individuals in order to maintain their base-line weight. For this reason, patients with inflammatory bowel disease often lose weight because they are unable to keep up with their increased caloric requirements. Physicians must keep this in mind when prescribing a diet for patients with inflammatory bowel disease, especially since malnourished patients are not as capable of maintaining their defense system (resistance) against infections and inflammation as individuals with adequate nutritional body stores.

BASIC FOOD GROUPS

Carbohydrates

Sugars and starches (carbohydrates) are composed of long chains of individual sugars linked by chemical bonds. Each gram of any sugar supplies 4 calories when metabolized by the body. In order to be absorbed and later utilized, the long chains of sugar must be broken down into their individual sugars within the small intestine. Enzymes released from the salivary glands and pancreas act on the chains of sugar molecules and break these down into the individual sugars, which then can be absorbed across the intestinal lining cells into the bloodstream. Each different type of carbohydrate is split by a separate enzyme. For instance, honey is composed mainly of simple glucose, which can be readily absorbed without the need for additional enzyme action. Table sugar (sucrose), on the other hand, is composed of two monosaccharide units (glucose and fructose) which require separation by the enzyme sucrase present in the surface lining of the intestine. Likewise, lactose, the sugar present in milk, is composed of glucose attached to galactose and requires the enzyme lactase for separation and later absorption. Starches are composed of much longer chains of glucose and require several different enzymes from the pancrease (amylase), which initially break the long chains into shorter chains that can be further divided by the enzymes along the intestinal lining.

Once absorbed into the bloodstream, all simple sugars are either converted to carbon dioxide, water, and energy or stored in the liver as glycogen for use at a later time. Relatively few steps are required to digest and absorb sugar as well as to metabolize the simple sugars into energy or a storage form. For this reason, sugars often provide a "quick" form of energy readily available to most individuals.

The ability to absorb sugars and starches thus depends on the integrity of the small intestine and, especially, the innermost lining, which contains the enzymes needed to break down and absorb the simple short chains of sugars. The pancreas also is necessary to convert the longer starch chains into shorter chains, which are then dealt with by the intestinal lining. Absorption of sugars is impaired when large segments of the small intestine are inflamed (as in Crohn's disease) or missing (as would occur after surgical removal of large segments of small intestines) and in the presence of over-growth of bacteria in the small bowel, which compete for the sugars and metabolize them for their own uses [as may occur in Crohn's disease when there is impairment of small intestinal motility (peristalsis) with partial obstruction or even the presence of a damaged (or absent) ileocecal valve, which allows backflow of bacteria from the colon into the ileum].

When, for any reason, sugars are not absorbed in the small intestine, they pass into the colon where the normal bacterial inhabitants metabolize (ferment) them into gas and small acids. The result is a combination of bloating and increased flatus accompanied by looser bowel movements and diarrhea as the unabsorbed particles draw water into the stool (by osmosis). One common form of malabsorption occurs in the condition of lactose intolerance. Many individuals are genetically "programmed" to cease manufacturing the lactase enzyme as they age through childhood. In this situation, consumption of large amounts of milk lead to symptoms in many individuals without inflammatory bowel disease. In patients with inflammatory bowel disease, the symptoms often are exaggerated because of the preexisting irritability of the gut and thus may be misinterpreted as active inflammatory disease.

The ability to digest lactose can be measured by simple tests. One method involves drinking a known quantity of lactose and then measuring the amount of sugar in the bloodstream. A simpler procedure measures the amount of hydrogen gas produced by intestinal bacteria whenever lactose is not absorbed. After swallowing the lactose, the patient exhales (breathes) into a bag at specific intervals, and the amount of hydrogen released by the breath correlates with the quantity of undigested sugar, in this case lactose. The latter examination is also a useful procedure to identify the presence of bacterial overgrowth of the small intestine, which might produce identical symptoms of diarrhea.

Not as well recognized is the fact that bulk or fiber derived from plant products also is composed of simple sugars identical to those in starches but linked by a different chemical bond. The human species (unlike certain bacteria) is not endowed with an effective enzyme capable of breaking down the bonds of fiber products, so the simple sugars are unavailable for absorption. In an undigested form, the fiber material remains within the large intestine and acts by an osmotic effect to retain water in the stool, producing a softer and more bulky bowel movement. However, a certain proportion of fiber is metabolized by the colonic bacteria. These bacteria are capable of splitting some of the bonds, creating numerous smaller particles (sugars) in the colon. The colon is not very efficient at absorbing the sugars, and subsequently, the bacteria further convert the sugars into their fermentation products of gas and acids, thus creating even more small particles. This explains why many patients develop bloating and sometimes diarrhea when they increase the amount of roughage in their diet.

Proteins

Just as starches are composed of long chains of sugars connected to one another by chemical bonds, proteins are composed of chains of amino acids. Each gram of protein or amino acid releases 4 calories of energy. Although most individuals do not realize that protein is an equivalent energy source to carbohydrates, the differences relate to how the foods are utilized by the body. Proteins are the main building blocks for muscle and can be either metabolized into simple sugars or incorporated into other proteins, which are incorporated into muscle and other body tissues.

Most of our protein sources are derived from animal products (meats of all kind, milk products, and eggs) as well as from some plants (soybeans). Similarly to carbohydrates, proteins also must be broken down into the smaller amino acids, which can then be absorbed from the small intestine into the bloodstream. In order to accomplish this, large amounts of protein must be ground and lubricated by teeth and saliva into a mixture that is further broken down within the stomach by acid and pepsin into long chains of amino acids. In the small intestine, these chains are further digested by enzymes released from the pancreas, forming individual amino acids, which then are able to pass through the intestinal lining cells into the bloodstream.

The protein digestion process usually is very efficient and does not require specialized enzymes in the lining of the small intestine in order to adequately absorb the individual amino acids. Abnormalities of protein absorption occur more commonly in individuals with abnormalities of the mouth (absence of teeth), stomach (inadequate acid production), or pancreas than in individuals with small intestinal defects. However, with severe inflammation or shortening of the small intestine, protein may not be adequately absorbed, and in extensive inflammation, protein actually can "weep" out into the bowel and be lost in the diarrheal stool. Protein deficiency complicating inflammatory bowel disease usually is attributed to diminished appetite reducing the intake of protein to levels below proper requirements, often as a consequence of the abdominal pain. Hence, an inadequate intake rather than impaired absorption accounts for most instances of protein malnutrition in inflammatory bowel disease.

Fats

The composition of fats is more complicated than that of carbohydrates or proteins. Fats are composed of three chains of fatty acids connected to a backbone of glycerol, forming what is known as a triglyceride. Fats are more energy efficient, providing 9 calories per gram, but they also require a more complicated process of absorption. Fats do not dissolve well in the intestine and require the presence of bile salts from the liver in order to mix with intestinal juices. Additionally, fats need the enzyme lipase produced in the pancreas to separate the individual fatty acids from the glycerol backbone. Along the small intestine these fatty acids are absorbed into the intestinal lining cell, reformed into triglycerides within the cells, and transported through the lymphatic system into the bloodstream.

The bile salts are then delivered to the terminal ileum, where they are absorbed and recycled into the bloodstream, collected in the liver, and circulated back to the bowel at the appropriate time to again mix with and make soluble fats in the small bowel.

Defective absorption of fats is a complication of liver or pancreatic disease, of intestinal inflammation which impairs the absorption of fatty acids, or of the absence of the terminal ileum, where bile salts are lost and cannot recirculate. The last situation produces an inadequate mixing of fats such that the pancreatic lipase cannot split the fatty acids, resulting in a loss of fat into the stool.

In Crohn's disease, the inflammation in the small intestine may impair absorption of the fatty acids, and disease or surgical removal of the terminal ileum can reduce the total availability of bile salts. Diarrhea may then occur for three reasons: if there are not sufficient bile salts to mix with fats, or if the fatty acids cannot be completely absorbed, these products are then transported into the colon where the normal colonic bacteria will break down the remaining triglycerides or long-chain fatty acids into short-chain fatty acids, which are irritants to the colon and can cause diarrhea. Similarly, with disease or absence of the terminal ileum, bile salts also will be transported into the colon and there converted into bile acids, which have a similar effect of producing diarrhea. These processes can occur together or independently, and they are differentiated by measuring the output of stool and the amount of fat in the stool over a 3-day period. If there are large amounts of fat in the stool, then the diarrhea may be improved by reducing the consumption of long-chain fats. This can be accomplished by avoiding highly fatty foods and greasy foods and by supplementing the diet with more easily absorbed fatty acids, medium-chain triglycerides, which do not require bile salts for absorption. If, on the other hand, there is no excessive elevation of fat, then one can assume that bile salts are the culprit, and a resin (cholestyramine) may be administered on a regular basis to bind the bile salts and prevent their conversion into bile acids by the colonic bacteria.

Thus, in presence of weight loss or diarrhea in inflammatory bowel disease, it is important to consult a physican who understands diet and nutrition further aided by a dietician/nutritionist to prescribe a diet that will be nutritious and yet not aggravate the symptoms of inflammatory bowel disease. Sometimes a few simple tests, as described above, will help to define the most appropriate dietary measures needed to insure adequate calories and weight gain and yet minimize the individual's symptoms.

Minerals

Although most people pay little attention to salts and minerals, these compounds are abundant in most foods and drinks that we consume and constitute a major portion of the body's chemicals. Sodium and chloride (salt) are the major constituents of all body fluids, and potassium is the major salt within the individual body cells. These chemicals are in constant balance and shift between the tissues and fluids (blood and secretions). The balance is maintained by an equilibrium between the amount of chemicals absorbed through the intestines and those excreted, mainly in the kidney and in the stool. Although we pay little attention to the amounts of these chemicals that we eat or drink, body mechanisms of thirst and fullness are directly linked to the internal levels of these important chemicals. Furthermore, little attention need to be paid to them, because the kidney is very efficient in both conserving and eliminating these salts so that a balance is virtually always maintained, except under the conditions of abnormally low intake, excessive tissue losses (diarrhea), or impairment of the elimination functions (kidney failure).

Diarrhea is one of the most common causes of imbalances of body salts. Both sodium and potassium accompany the fluid loss resulting in imbalances leading to dehydration (loss of sodium) or muscle weakness and irritability (with the loss of potassium). Some of these abnormalities can be determined by the physician by evaluating differences in blood pressure between lying and standing, testing the resiliency (turgor) of the skin, examining muscle strength and reflexes and, most reliably, by simple blood determinations of levels of serum electrolytes (sodium, potassium, chloride, and bicarbonate).

Calcium is an important mineral and the major component of

bone. Calcium compounds provide the hardness and strength of bone, and blood and tissue levels are closely controlled by a combination of factors. Absorption of calcium from the gut is facilitated by the presence of vitamin D. Vitamin D, a fat-soluble vitamin, is absorbed in the terminal ileum and converted into its active form by both the liver and kidney. A significant proportion of vitamin D is actually produced in the skin after conversion of the inactive form into the active form by sunlight. Deficiencies of vitamin D and/or inadequate exposure to sunlight may cause insufficient absorption of calcium to maintain the bone strength. This condition, called osteomalacia, develops in Crohn's disease when severe involvement or surgical absence of the terminal ileum leads to vitamin D deficiency.

Blood levels of calcium are regulated by a hormone produced in four small glands near the thyroid gland in the neck (parathyroids). Parathyroid hormone maintains the balance of calcium between the blood and bone and controls the elimination of calcium in the kidneys. Deficiencies of the parathyroid glands will cause low serum calcium, whereas overactivity can produce high serum calcium. When the calcium levels in the blood are low, the muscles become irritable and twitch or contract vigorously (tetanus); with high levels of calcium, muscular activity is reduced and may be associated with fatigue and constipation.

Magnesium is another mineral intricately related to calcium. Magnesium also is important in the regulation of calcium as well as in many cellular functions. Severe diarrhea can cause a lowering of the serum magnesium, which causes a secondary loss of serum calcium through the kidneys. Magnesium deficiency also is manifested as irritability of the muscles and may lead to seizures.

Phosphorus, a mineral found in many plants, is essential for bone production as well as for many of the cellular enzyme systems. Diarrhea can also cause a leaching of the phosphate with symptoms of generalized weakness, difficulty in swallowing, and, in severe cases, heart failure.

Iron is an essential mineral for the formation of red blood cells and muscles. Iron deficiency is one of the more commonly encountered mineral disorders in inflammatory bowel disease and occurs in any condition accompanied by bleeding in which the blood loss is greater than the intake of iron. Anemia secondary to inadequate iron stores is often noted in women with excessive menstrual bleeding.

Intestinal bleeding is such a common problem in patients with inflammatory bowel disease that iron deficiency is probably the most frequent nutritional deficit. Anemia is the usual symptom and may become manifest as fatigue, weakness, or, in extreme situations, shortness of breath. Many patients will require replacement therapy by one of three routes.

Iron pills taken by mouth may cause additional gastrointestinal upset. To prevent this problem, the tablets should be spaced throughout the day and may be consumed with meals. Multiple injections of iron can be given into the muscles, but this requires a deep injection, which is often painful and can cause a permanent discoloration of the skin. Finally, iron may be administered via an intravenous drip over several hours. This last method is rarely complicated by allergic reactions or a delayed onset of "flu-like" symptoms of fevers, muscle or joint pains, or rashes. Options related to iron replacement should be discussed with one's physician and depend on the individual's symptoms and tolerance of oral iron products.

Diarrhea is the most common mechanism whereby the abovementioned body minerals are lost in inflammatory bowel disease. Controlling the inflammation is the most effective way of preventing and reversing these losses. Some individuals with severe losses secondary to an intestinal tract shortened by surgery require additional mineral replacements either in the diet or via intramuscular or intravenous injections. Under most circumstances. these deficiencies are easily diagnosed by blood tests in patients suspected of having excess mineral loss because of watery stools. On rare occasions, an individual will come to a physician's attention for the consequences of mineral deficiencies rather than the diarrhea itself.

Trace Elements

Many chemicals are needed by the body in very small amounts in order to act as "cofactors" necessary for enzyme or metabolic systems. Although required in minute amounts, these chemicals are essential for life, and deficiencies can cause severe reactions. Trace elements include zinc, manganese, copper, and cobalt among others. Dietary inadequacies are rare except in extraordinary circumstances of severe protracted diarrhea or highly artificial diets. Zinc deficiency has been recognized in patients with Crohn's disease complicated by significant diarrhea and may lead to anemia and diabetes. Such conditions are relatively rare but occur in patients with the most severe symptoms. Other deficiencies of trace elements have only been described in patients with virtually no oral food intake who are receiving all of their nutrition by intravenous feeding. The accompanying diarrhea may worsen the inadequacies through excessive losses in the stool. Only now are we learning how to measure such deficiencies.

Vitamins

Vitamins are more complex chemicals required as regulators of many body processes. They do not actually produce energy but are important for biochemical reactions and cellular functions. Vitamins are divided into categories according to the manner in which they are absorbed by the intestines. These relate to their ability to dissolve in water or fat.

Water-soluble vitamins are absorbed throughout the small intestines and include the B vitamins, vitamin C, folic acid, and others. Significant deficiencies of the water-soluble vitamins have been described in severe Crohn's disease. Rarely, symptoms of skin rashes, a shiny or glossy tongue, diarrhea, or nerve damage may be related to deficiencies of the B vitamins. Excess ingestion of some of the B vitamins and niacin can produce diarrhea, flushing, and palpitations.

Vitamic C deficiency may lead to cracking of the corners of the mouth, poor wound healing, or deformity of the bones as in scurvy. The role of vitamin C as pertains to the immune system and resistance to infections remains controversial. Vitamin C deficiency is *not* known to predispose to infections, yet, as has been popularized in the lay press, large quantities of vitamin C have been shown in a few studies to prevent viral infections in selected groups of patients. Less well advertised are the numerous reports that have not been able to confirm the original investigation. We tend to follow a more conservative approach to the issue. Small doses of vitamin C are unlikely to be harmful; however, large quantities (over 1,000 mg) can cause gastric and intestinal irritation, acidification of the urine, and may predispose patients to the formation of oxalate kidney stones.

Folic acid is important for growth of nerves, red blood cells, and intestinal lining cells (epithelium); deficiency may result from poor dietary intake or damage to the intestine or be related to impaired absorption in the presence of sulfasalazine. As mentioned previously, individuals taking significant doses of sulfasalazine should also receive supplementary folic acid.

Vitamin B_{12} also is a water-soluble vitamin absorbed exclusively by the terminal ileum. In addition, vitamin B_{12} requires a chemical produced by the stomach (intrinsic factor) for conversion into a form recognized by special receptors in the terminal ileum. Damage to the stomach as in pernicious anemia, longstanding gastritis, or surgery will impair the ability to absorb vitamin B_{12}. Likewise, inflammatory damage or surgical absence of the terminal ileum, both of which are common in Crohn's disease, will limit the amount of vitamin B_{12} that can be absorbed. This vitamin is essential for the formation of blood cells and nerves, and a chronic deficiency will produce anemia and/or nerve damage. The serum levels of vitamin B_{12} can be measured by simple blood tests, and, at times, the physician may wish to evaluate the ability to absorb vitamin B_{12} by mouth with a Schilling's test. Here, the vitamin is "labeled" with a minute radioactive marker and is administered by mouth and measured in the urine. In cases in which absorption is inadequate because of ileal disease or surgery, replacement of vitamin B_{12} by supplemental intramuscular injections may become a lifelong requirement.

Fat-Soluble Vitamins

The fat-soluble vitamins (vitamins A, D, E, and K) also require a healthy terminal ileum for effective absorption. This is because of the importance of the ileum for bile salt and fat absorption, as previously discussed. Vitamin A is essential for light receptors in the retina of the eye, and deficiency of Vitamin A leads to night blindness, abnormalities of the cornea (or outer coating of the eye), and dry, scaly skin. Vitamin D is essential for calcium balance and bone formation. Vitamin E is required by the body in very small amounts and is significantly reduced in only the most extreme cases of Crohn's disease. Vitamin E probably is important for nerve growth, although only few vitamin E deficiency conditions have been described. Vitamin K is actually produced by the normal bacterial inhabitants of the gut and is lowered in patients who take frequent antibiotics for long periods of time without adequate supplementation of vitamin K and in patients with significant ileal disease or fat malabsorption. Vitamin K is essential for blood clotting, and deficiencies of vitamin K will produce easy bruisability and a bleeding tendency often manifest as bleeding of the gums while brushing teeth or as excessive menstruation.

Since Crohn's disease often affects the terminal ileum, measured levels of vitamins A, D, E, and K are often low, and supplementation by additional vitamins in the diet or, rarely, by intramuscular injection may become necessary.

DIET THERAPY IN INFLAMMATORY BOWEL DISEASE

No specific diet will be correct for all patients with inflammatory bowel disease; individual needs are more important. The recommendations regarding the diet depend on individual symptoms, the location of the inflammation, previous surgery, or complications such as strictures, fissures, or perianal disease (hemorrhoids and fissures). Again, no diet is known to cause or worsen the *inflammation* of inflammatory bowel disease; however, alterations in one's diet may significantly influence *symptoms*.

An example of how dietary modifications apply to different sets of patients is that of roughage (fiber). As described above, fiber products consist of the undigested portion of plants and include a variety of different compounds (e.g., cellulose, pectins, lignins, gums), all of which function to some degree by adding bulk and retained water within the stool. However, it is easy to recognize how different forms of roughage may be tolerated to variable degrees by individual patients. For instance, fresh fruits and vegetables are more laxative than cooked (or canned) products, and a major proportion of this effect is derived from skins. Hence, for patients with a tendency towards diarrhea, it is reasonable to limit the consumption of fresh fruits and vegetables in favor of cooked, canned, or peeled produce. On the other hand, for patients who are constipated (for example with mild proctitis), increasing the portions of fruits and vegetables in the diet may be quite useful. In these and most cases of inflammatory bowel disease, one must also recognize that, aside from their laxative properties, fresh fruit and vegetable roughage may be irritating to an inflamed bowel as the coarse grains rub against an ulcerated, congested segment of intestine. Furthermore, nuts and seeds are poorly digested and may scrape inflamed areas, causing bleeding or, along with residues of other undigested fiber (e.g, celery), block (obstruct) narrowed or strictured loops of bowel.

We usually caution against the intake of nuts, seeds, corn, and popcorn for the reasons just mentioned. A common analogy is peanuts and peanut butter. Peanut butter is totally acceptable because it is in a modified form that will not block the bowel. Peanuts, on the other hand, if not chewed to a pulp, can pass through the digestive tract unaltered and can potentially become caught in a narrowed segment or irritate an inflamed or friable segment of the bowel lining.

Highly spiced foods are irritants to the bowel and cause frequent and/or painful bowel movements in healthy individuals without inflammatory bowel disease. This effect results from the activation of nerve fibers in the bowel stimulating motility. In most patients with inflammatory bowel disease, highly seasoned foods should be avoided. We also often restrict the amounts of fruit juices, especially citrus fruits, because of the concentrated load of sugars, which may not be fully digested within the bowel and can cause gas and diarrhea. Also, highly fatty or greasy foods may also be incompletely absorbed and can cause diarrhea.

In general, a "middle-of-the-road" diet is most reasonable for patients with any abdominal symptoms. We suggest that individuals adjust their intake of fruits and vegetables according to their bowel habits. To maintain regular, formed stools, most normal persons will require between four and six servings of fruits and/or vegetables daily. For constipation, the portions are increased; for diarrhea, cooked, canned, or peeled products are more suitable. Avoiding the extremes of highly seasoned, highly fatty or greasy, and highly sweetened foods is reasonable. *Certain patients should eliminate any food items that they individually find intolerable or that reliably produce symptoms.*

For any individual with inflammatory bowel disease, it is also important that their physician review their dietary habits to make certain that no essential food groups are missing. The doctor can further adjust the diet to maximize relief of symptoms and supplement with appropriate calories, protein, minerals, or vitamins to avoid significant deficiencies. Consultation by dietician or nutritionist is essential for many patients, especially those with significant weight loss, diarrhea, vomiting, or intermittent blockage of the bowel. These experts may identify a previously unrecognized nutritional deficit and can replace or substitute dietary equivalents for prescribed exclusions (e.g., calcium substitutes for patients who are lactose intolerant and must avoid milk products).

SPECIFIC DIETARY THERAPIES

Some patients may temporarily require radical alterations of eating patterns to the point of completely liquid diets. These may be recommended to give the bowel a partial rest in patients with difficult to control diarrhea, severe cramps, intermittent blockage, or fistulas. The elimination of all residue (fiber and roughage) allows the bowel to absorb virtually all essential nutrients while producing minimal amounts of stool. Less material will then be transported to the ileum and colon, thus reducing the work load of these organs, allowing the distal bowel to rest. With the availability of completely nutritious liquid food supplements, such diets are now possible. Although somewhat more costly than regular food items, these products offer the potential for at-home therapy and the avoidance of more drastic medical therapy (complete intravenous, or i.v., feeding, see the following discussion), the ability to reduce medications, and the possible cancellation of anticipated surgery. When recommendations for such a diet are necessary, a complete dietary evaluation and consultation with a dietician is essential.

HYPERALIMENTATION

Hyperalimentation (total parenteral nutrition, TPN) is a method of feeding the patient totally by means of a vein. Such therapy may be necessary for those people who are unable to eat for long periods of time because of symptoms, severe illness, or surgery. Additional indications for hyperalimentation include nutritional restoration for severely malnourished patients in general or those anticipating surgery, as treatment for an inflammatory mass or certain fistulas, or to reverse growth retardation in children. Hyperalimentation and bowel rest also may be beneficial in controlling the symptoms of inflammatory bowel disease while replenishing weight and stores of calories, protein, fat, vitamins, and minerals. The hyperalimentation itself provides the necessary calories and nutrients to replenish the body losses, yet the concept of bowel rest implies much more.

The gut is an immune-system organ that is constantly bombarded by foods, drugs, toxins, and microorganisms. An elaborate array of immune cells lines the gastrointestinal tract, which must discriminate between the compounds required for absorption and potentially harmful substances. With intestinal inflammation, this barrier is disrupted, and the local immune system must contend with more than usual exposure to the gut contents. When "rest" eliminates further exposure of the gut to multiple antigens, inflammatory responsive cells that are already "turned on" by the underlying disease can avoid further activation, and the inflammatory reaction subsides. Furthermore, the ingestion of food stimulates both intestinal secretion of acid and enzymes and heightened motility of the smooth musculature. In the setting of intestinal inflammation and the accompanying heightened sensitivity to normal stimuli, reducing the activity of the gut provides it with relief from symptoms (abdominal pain, diarrhea, etc.) and an opportunity to repair itself. The improvement in the nutritional state also intensifies the body's ability to heal infections.

We can now provide almost unlimited calories by vein, which makes it possible to feed the most severely malnourished individuals. More than 2,000 calories can now be given daily through a regular intravenous catheter, although specialized feeding lines are more commonly placed into larger veins in the shoulder underneath the collarbone (subclavian) or in the neck (jugular) (Fig. 10). The advantage of placing a larger-bore catheter into the ''central'' veins is that more calories can be given throughout the day since the administered fluids are rapidly diluted by the greater blood flow in the bigger veins. Such feedings may be continuously administered over 24 hours through an infusion pump, or, after some period of adjustment, all of the fluid and nutrition needed can be administered overnight so that the i.v. can be unhooked during the day if a specialized catheter (Hickman) has been used.

Some patients who require long-term (weeks, months, years, and rarely, life-long) treatment with complete intravenous hyperalimentation can be treated at home. With more hyperalimentation, individuals learn to prepare a portion of their i.v. feedings for self-

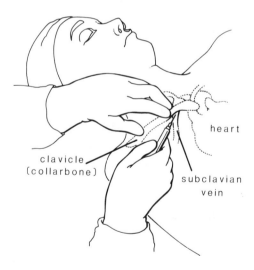

FIG. 10. Insertion of hyperalimentation (TPN) catheter into the subclavian vein.

administration during an in-hospital training period. After "gradua-tion," they can be discharged to home where they can infuse the feedings overnight while they are sleeping. In the morning, they can unhook the "lines" with meticulous care and sanitation (sterile technique) and then go off to work or school during the day. We have had patients who are capable of some sports activities (golf, jogging, and even tennis) when these lines have been in place. In patients with severely damaged bowel or bowel that is greatly short-ened because of multiple operations, hyperalimentation is the only means by which they can have sufficient calories to survive. Until the time that intestinal transplants become available, hyperalimenta-tion remains a true lifeline yet allows individuals to live an other-wise normal existence.

Long-term hyperalimentation is a dramatic approach that is, at the present time, reserved for the most troublesome or complicated cases. There is no question that this therapy requires an even greater adjustment for individuals who already have had to adapt to a long-standing physical ailment with constant negative emotional impact. The cost of such therapy is also extraordinary. Nevertheless, one must weigh these factors against the potential gain from this approach, which, at minimum provides relief from chronically per-sisting symptoms and has the potential for reducing the dosage of corticosteroids and avoiding (additional) surgery.

It must be emphasized that the methods of assessing nutritional requirements and of prescribing the appropriate diet require a team of professionals that includes a physician, a nutritionist, a pharma-cist, and a nurse who, together, are able to implement, adjust, and maintain the necessary dietary constituents and materials needed for long-term nutritional therapy. Rarely can a single physician or other individual provide all the supports necessary for the maintenance and monitoring of hyperalimentation (and especially home hyperalimentation), and a patient should be wary of any physician or group that prescribes TPN without the availability of such a nutrition support team.

CHAPTER 10

Surgical Therapy

ULCERATIVE COLITIS

Ulcerative colitis, in an ultimate sense, is a curable disease. The definitive cure involves removal of the entire colon and rectum. Unfortunately, to date, the most reliable (uncomplicated) method of achieving this cure usually requires the formation of an ileostomy (Fig. 11). This involves surgical removal of the entire colon, rectum, and anus with a surgical closure of the crease between the buttocks. The last portion of the ileum is brought through an opening in the skin of the abdominal wall and sutured down to the skin. This opening, or stoma, is then surrounded by an appliance to collect the drainage. The drainage consists of small bowel contents (unabsorbed food and bile), which do not have the feculent qualities of stool since the bacterial population of the small intestine is limited and formation of feces or stool by putrefaction does not occur. Hence, the contents remain fluid (although sometimes thickened) and do not have the odor of stool.

After such an operation, virtually all patients regain their health. There is no chance of recurrence of true ulcerative colitis, and the individual can lead an entirely normal life. There are essentially no limitations to his or her activities including occupation, sports (except violent contact sports), sex, or childbearing capabilities. Follow-up medical care returns to yearly routine examinations. No medications are required, and the life expectancy is that of an individual who has never had ulcerative colitis.

117

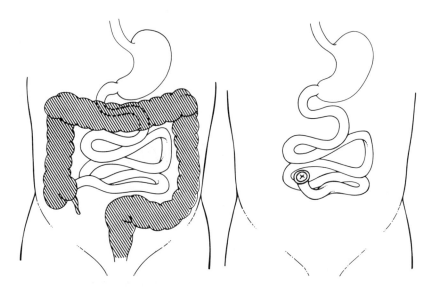

FIG. 11. Colectomy **(left)** and ileostomy **(right)**.

Indications for Surgery

The reasons for operating on an individual with ulcerative colitis are well defined. The most urgent reason for an operation is a toxic megacolon that does not rapidly respond (within 48 to 72 hr) to medical treatment. In this situation, the wall of the colon becomes tissue-paper thin, and the entire large bowel may dilate, risking perforation of the bowel. This complication requires an emergency operation. Uncontrollable bleeding is another reason for performing emergency surgery.

The development of cancer or persistent, severe dysplasia within the colon also warrants a colectomy. In either of these situations, total removal of the colon and rectum is recommended to eliminate completely any possibility of future large bowel cancers. Another indication for an operation might be a stricture, or strictures that interfere with colonic function or appear highly suspicious of harboring a malignancy (cancer).

Less well-defined indications for surgery require the joint participation of the patient and physician in the decision of the appropriate timing of an operation. One such situation would be for persistent, undesirable side effects of medications (e.g., corticosteroids), where many adverse effects may be intolerable to the patient. Such adverse effects include the formation of cataracts, thinning of the bones, changes of the skin, maldistribution of fat, as well as the possibility of developing diabetes. If any of these situations occurs, then an individual may prefer to have an operation than to continue complicated medical treatment and an uncertain outcome.

An even more debatable indication for surgery involves the "failure to respond to medical treatment." This usually means that a patient has become dissatisfied with the limitations imposed by chronic colitis on his or her life-style, family, job, or interests. Frequent bowel movements, occasional loss of bowel control, side effects of medication, the expense of medication, or simply frustration over the unpredictably variable course of a chronic illness can overwhelm an individual and lead that patient to request an operation. At this point, the rapport between the physician and the patient and family becomes very important so that the right decision can be made. A complete understanding of the options involved is critical, for once an operation has been performed, it is not reversible, and the decision is one the patient will have to live with for the rest of his or her life. In our experience, when the decision is well thought out and the options are completely understood, the great majority of individuals are able to look forward to and lead happy, well-fulfilled lives.

Surgical Alternatives

One question that frequently arises during the consideration of surgery for ulcerative colitis is whether only the diseased portion of the colon can be removed. Often when the rectum appears less diseased or if a portion of the colon is spared from active inflammation, the patient or his family will ask, and reasonably so, "Why can't that portion be saved?" and the possibility of bowel continuity and anal continence (the ability to pass bowel movements through the healthy rectum and anus) be preserved. As a matter of fact, some surgeons will perform just such an operation if the rectum is not severely involved.

Although this remains a controversial alternative, it does not eliminate the need for continued treatment of the ulcerative colitis. In other words, the inflammatory process can continue in the portion of the colon that has been retained, and all of the previously mentioned medical means of treatment may be necessary to control the colitis. Additionally, the risk of developing dysplasia or cancer remains, and it is necessary to perform regular proctoscopic or colonoscopic examinations at intervals to make certain that a cancer or precancer is not developing. Also, with a portion of the colon removed, the bowel movements will be more liquid and more numerous. In other cases, the previously controlled inflammation may worsen to the point that medical therapy needs to be intensified, or a second operation may ultimately be required to control the inflammation. Hence, we rarely recommend such a procedure for the great majority of our patients. In a few individuals, a partial removal of the colon may be possible, and in these circumstances a very lengthy discussion outlining all of the possible sequelae of a limited operation is warranted among the patient, the patient's family, the surgeon, and the gastroenterologist caring for the patient. This rarely is an acceptable solution to the problem of ulcerative colitis.

Colectomy and Ileostomy

The standard operation involves a total removal of the colon and rectum with the formation of an ileostomy. In recent decades, this operation has been perfected so that previously encountered complications of ileostomies (poor wound healing, leakage, and poor functioning of the stoma) can be avoided. The operation itself may be lengthy (at times lasting 6 to 10 hours), but in competent hands it has become routine. The operation is performed through an incision in the abdominal wall, and the surgeon will then remove the entire colon through the abdomen. Removal of the rectum requires repositioning the patient on the operating table, and the surgeon works from below the buttocks to carefully separate the tissues of the rectum from the surrounding structures (the bladder and the prostate in men, the vagina in women). After removal of the colon and rectum, the end of the small intestine is brought through a separate opening in the abdomen and is then closed onto the skin, leaving a small stub protruding approximately ½ inch above the skin line. The ileostomy appliance is then placed around the stomal opening for collection of the intestinal output.

After such an operation, most patients awaken with a tube protruding from their nose (a nasogastric tube), which drains the stomach and prevents the nausea and vomiting that may occur while the bowel is paralyzed for a period of time after the operation. The doctors listen to the abdomen daily for the return of bowel activity, which is heralded by the output of fluid or gas into the ileostomy bag. At that time, the nasogastric tube is usually removed, and shortly thereafter the patient begins on liquid feedings, which are gradually advanced over several days to solids. The postoperative recovery time is usually between 1 and 2 weeks in the hospital followed by another week or two at home with gradually progressive activities. By 4 to 6 weeks after the operation, the patient can expect to be in excellent health and to have regained virtually all his or her strength.

The operation itself usually proceeds smoothly. Although uncommon, a few potential adverse consequences may arise. Occasionally, the newly formed ileostomy may not function well and become swollen and at times blocked. This may lead to a somewhat longer period of nasogastric tube suctioning or an interval of refeeding. There is also the possibility that scar tissue (adhesions) may form after any operation, which can lead to a bowel obstruction some time after the surgery. The latter can occur anywhere from days to years after the operation and may cause abdominal pain, vomiting, and decreased output through the stoma. This problem requires the placement of a nasogastric tube to decompress the blockage that occurs when the bowel twists around an adhesion and becomes swollen and the channel narrowed. By removing the bowel contents through the tube above the obstruction, the bowel can decompress and regain its normal size. Eventually, the swelling is allowed to reduce such that, in many cases, the normal flow can return. At times, however, an additional operation is necessary to free the twisted intestine if it becomes in danger of losing its blood supply, which would cause that loop of bowel to die. Again, we must emphasize that this complication is uncommon.

Other rare complications of the conventional ileostomy include urinary difficulties or, in men, the inability to maintain an erection. These problems are caused by the proximity of the nerves supplying the bladder and penis to the wall of the rectum. During the operation, the surgeon must carefully separate the rectal tissue from these nerves, but at times the tissue damage or swelling from the operation itself may cause injury and produce a temporary or rarely permanent dysfunction. In order to prevent urinary distention after the operation, a catheter is kept in place between 5 to 10 days after the surgery, until the bladder regains its proper function.

During the postoperative period, the patient is given instructions as to how to operate, clean, and care for the stoma so that by the time he or she returns home, he or she will be comfortable dealing with the new system. The great majority of individuals adapt quite well to their new body function, and most hospitals provide additional counseling through an enterostomal nurse. Over the years, most patients will develop their own system of caring for the appliance and learn individual "tricks" of style for living with the ostomy (see Chapter 13).

Surgical Alternatives

Several new techniques are currently under development that may ultimately provide better choices for the ulcerative colitis patient when surgery is recommended. There currently are two different types of investigational surgical approaches that are available in a few centers around the country and abroad. It must be remembered that these procedures have only been used for a relatively short period of time and that the long-term outcomes have not yet been fully determined.

The first procedure is called a continent ileostomy or Koch's pouch (Fig. 12A). In this procedure, the entire colon and rectum are removed as described above. However, instead of bringing the last portion of the ileum out to the surface, the ileum is folded over itself beneath the abdominal wall, and an internal pouch is created with a

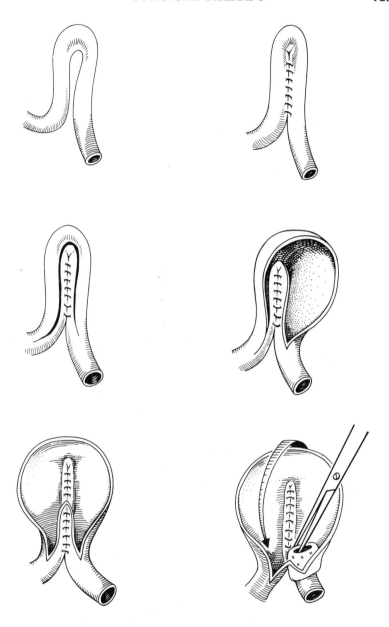

FIG. 12A. Formation of ileal reservoir.

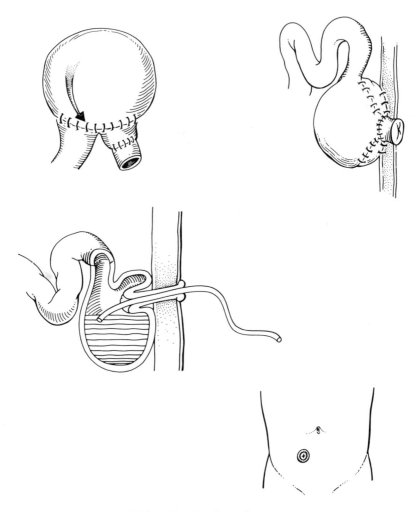

FIG. 12B. Continent ileostomy.

small nipple valve opening to the surface (Fig. 12B). The internal
pouch acts as a reservoir to collect the intestinal drainage, and the
nipple valve prevents uncontrolled expulsion of the liquid contents.
To empty the reservoir, a small tube or catheter is placed through
the nipple valve, and the pouch can be drained on a regular schedule
throughout the day or as needed.

The concept of an internal reservoir is very satisfying, especially for individuals who are intensely concerned about their body image and who do not feel that they could emotionally accept the external appliance. At the present time, however, there are several problems with this technique.

To begin with, the creation of the internal pouch will usually require a second surgical procedure after the abdominal colectomy. This is because of the necessity of providing a temporary stoma to drain stool as the pouch is "maturing." Eventually, the stoma is closed, and the pouch becomes functional. Additionally, the optimal technique for creating such a pouch has not yet been determined. Many patients have had to undergo numerous operations for revisions of the internal pouch because it either leaked or did not empty properly and became obstructed. We are aware of some patients who have undergone at least a dozen reoperations and whose pouch has still not functioned adequately. Another basic problem that has yet to be fully worked out is that the small intestine has not evolved to perform the function of a reservoir. The normal lining of the small intestine is quite different from that of the colon and, when exposed to stagnant contents, can become inflamed, a condition referred to as "pouchitis." In this situation, the patient may develop new inflammatory symptoms such as fever, diarrhea, intestinal bleeding, and abdominal pain. In many instances, this problem will respond to a course of antibiotics. However, the best means of preventing and treating pouchitis over long periods of time has not yet been fully elucidated. Some patients have required a reversal of the continent ileostomy to the standard ileostomy for the treatment of one of the above complications.

The continent ileostomy appears to be most effective in a small proportion of individuals, especially young women and thin patients. It is less well tolerated by older and overweight individuals. Because of the, as yet, unstandardized operative technique, we are reluctant to recommend this procedure for any but a select few.

A second novel surgical approach is known as the ileoanal anastomosis (Fig. 13). For this procedure, the colectomy is again performed as described for the standard technique. However, the

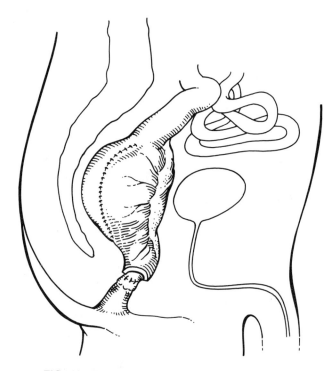

FIG. 13. Ileoanal anastomosis with ileal reservoir.

rectum is handled in a different manner. Instead of removing the entire rectum, the innermost lining (mucosa) is stripped away, preserving the underlying musculature. The ileum is then brought down and sewn into the surrounding sheath of rectal muscle. The rationale for this procedure is to maintain control of bowel movements, which are passed through the anus, and yet to remove the actively diseased rectal mucosa, which also carries the potential to become malignant over long periods of time. One typical addition to this procedure that has been developed in recent years has been the formation of an internal J-pouch created by several loops of the ileum so that the new rectum has some reservoir capacity, as described for the continent ileostomy.

When perfected, this may be the ideal technique for patients with ulcerative colitis confronted with the necessity of a colectomy. However, at the time of this writing, several problems remain with the technique. The most common difficulties arise during the initial period of adaptation to the surgery. Until the new ''rectum'' adapts, many individuals will pass 20 bowel movements through the day, some of which are associated with leakage or incontinence. Other patients may not be able to spontaneously pass the movements through the anus and require a tube to empty out the reservoir. Again, as with the continent ileostomy, the ideal technique for producing an internal reservoir has yet to be perfected. Also, one must keep in mind that the formation of this anastomosis will also require a second operation and at times a third. This procedure often calls for a temporary ileostomy to allow the new connection within the rectum to heal properly. Several weeks or months later, the stoma is closed so that the fecal stream again passes through the anus. As with the continent ileostomy, the ileum acting as a reservoir can become inflamed or obstructed and may require treatment with antibiotics or, if extreme, necessitate a final conversion to a standard ileostomy.

Experience with this technique has been most sucessful in younger individuals (children) and those who are extremely well motivated and willing to persevere through the initial months of frequent bowel movements, occasional leakage (especially at night), the possible necessity of wearing a diaper, and the need for several surgeries in order to make the procedure functional.

It is not certain what can be expected over long periods (years) of time after this procedure. We are aware that the lining of the rectum can become cancerous in ulcerative colitis, and, although it is theoretically removed, small patches may have been overlooked and would then retain the potential to cause future problems. We expect that this procedure will gain popularity over time and eventually become a reasonable alternative for many patients. However, at the present time, it must also be considered investigational and should be limited to those patients who are extremely well motivated and willing to undergo a 12-month period of adaptation to the new rectum.

CROHN'S DISEASE

Because of the variable location and complications of Crohn's disease, a description of the surgical possibilities is much more difficult than the clear-cut options available for ulcerative colitis. Additionally, it must be kept in mind that whereas ulcerative colitis is a disease curable by surgical resection, Crohn's disease is only palliated (treated symptomatically without the possibility of cure). After the involved segment of bowel is removed in Crohn's disease, there is a strong likelihood that the inflammation will recur, especially at the anastomotic site (the location where the bowel was reconnected). For this reason, we emphasize operating for symptoms and complications of Crohn's disease rather than viewing surgery as a primary or initial treatment.

There are, however, a number of definite indications for surgery in Crohn's disease. The first, and probably the most common need for surgery, arises in the presence of an obstruction. When the bowel becomes so narrowed that the intestinal contents cannot pass through, the patient will develop severe abdominal cramps and vomiting. In some instances the narrowing is only temporary, related to swelling (edema) in the location of the inflammation, and may respond to medical treatment alone. The patient will require a nasogastric tube to decompress (shrink) the bowel back to its original size by emptying the contents that are blocked. When this is successful, the swelling often reduces, and in many cases the bowel will open up again. If the obstruction is not relieved by medical treatment, then removal of that segment of bowel by an operation will be necessary. The surgeon will usually remove only the small segment of bowel that is most inflamed and then reconnect the two ends in what is called a "primary anastomosis." Rarely, in obstruction, there will be an associated abscess cavity or free pus inside the abdomen. It is also possible for the bowel to perforate (rupture), in which case intestinal contents can empty into the abdominal cavity and cause peritonitis. If either of these mentioned complications occur, it may not be possible to reconnect the bowel immediately because in these settings of inflammation or pus, the suture line (stitches) at the anastomosis is at risk of falling apart, and the connection will not hold. Therefore, a temporary ileostomy may be necessary, which can be reconnected at a second operation after a 6- to 12-week recovery period.

Another indication for surgery in Crohn's disease is the case of an abdominal mass, abscess, or fistula that does not respond to medical treatment. In these situations, it is more common to require a temporary ileostomy before the bowel can be reconnected. At surgery, the portion of the bowel that is most severely diseased (and leads to the complication) may be removed and the rest of the bowel left untouched.

Uncontrollable bleeding is an uncommon but often urgent complication that may require surgery in Crohn's disease. At the operation, the surgeon will identify the site of blood loss and usually only remove the involved segment of bowel.

As with ulcerative colitis, the "failure to respond to medical therapy" is a less well-defined indication for surgery in Crohn's disease. This may also be the case for patients who have had intolerable side effects of the medical therapy or if medical treatment with steroids cannot be reduced. In children, retardation of growth that does not respond to medical treatment emphasizing a liberal intake of calories and protein may also be an indication for the removal of the most severely inflamed segment of bowel.

Although surgery is a last resort in Crohn's disease, the response of the patient often is quite dramatic and beneficial. If all of the detectable inflammation is removed at the operation, it is usually possible to decrease and discontinue all medications. This outcome, depends on how much bowel is removed, how much bowel remains, the location of the bowel removed, and whether or not the remaining intestine is free of active inflammation.

If the patient has been on steroids prior to the operation, it will be necessary to reduce the dosage gradually in order to allow the adrenal gland to recover. Most individuals will find on discharge that they are on a fraction of their initial medication, and the majority will feel complete relief from their symptoms. When the appropriate surgical procedure has been timed to occur after a patient has been adequately prepared (nutritional deficiencies have been restored and supervening infections treated) one can anticipate an excellent outcome.

After the operation the patient usually awakens with a nasogastric tube in place to prevent nausea and vomiting and to protect the reconnected bowel from larger amounts of highly acidic stomach contents passing through and eroding the new connection (anastomosis). When bowel sounds return, as described for ulcerative colitis, the nasogastric tube can be withdrawn, and the patient will be gradually refed an enlarging diet. Usually this will begin with clear liquids, and over several days, soft and then solid foods can be added. The anticipated recovery period for uncomplicated surgery in Crohn's disease is approximately 1 to 2 weeks in the hospital and several more weeks of recuperation at home.

The exact surgical procedure for Crohn's disease will, of course, depend on the location of the disease and the particular problem requiring treatment. The most common operation involves removal of the terminal ileum and cecum (Fig. 14). The ileum is then reconnected to the ascending colon, as the ileocecal valve is lost. Patients may then find that they have a tendency towards more frequent and looser bowel movements even though there is an adequate length of colon to produce formed stools. The reason for this is that the ileocecal valve would normally slow down transport of the liquid small intestinal contents into the large bowel. When the valve is absent, the contents continuously drain into the colon, and it takes time for the remaining small intestine and the colon to adapt to this new system before it will produce formed stools.

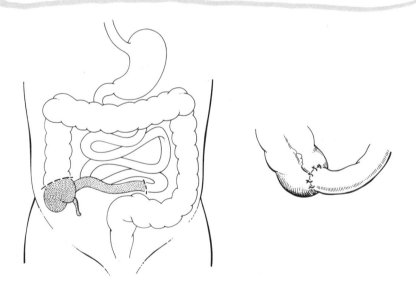

FIG. 14. Resection of ileum and cecum.

Some dietary adjustments may be helpful in preventing this form of diarrhea, including a reduction in fat intake (avoiding highly greasy and fried foods), since fats may not be completely absorbed in the ileum and can be converted to fatty acids, which stimulate colonic activity and fluid secretion. Reducing the roughage intake is also helpful in the initial adaptive postoperative interval, as the ingestion of bulk or fiber products will increase the number of bowel movements. Another measure that is often helpful when a large segment of the ileum has been removed may be the prescription of cholestyramine, a resin that binds to bile acids. Bile acids, like fatty acids, are normally absorbed in the terminal ileum. When a lengthy segment of ileum has been removed, the bile salts are incompletely absorbed and pass into the colon, where they are converted into bile acids by the bacteria and stimulate the bowel to secrete fluid, resulting in diarrhea. Discussions with a physician and or nutritionist may be useful in adjusting the diet after small intestinal surgery for Crohn's disease.

Surgery of the colon for Crohn's disease allows more options than exist for ulcerative colitis. When Crohn's disease involves the colon (Crohn's colitis or granulomatous colitis), a partial or complete removal of the colon is sometimes necessary. When the inflammation is limited to the colon and does not involve any portion of the small intestine, a total colectomy will be curative in the majority of patients, and the Crohn's disease will not recur in the small bowel if an ileostomy is created. On the other hand, when the disease involves the proximal or right colon alone and spares the rectum, it is often possible to connect the ileum directly to the rectum, thus preserving continuity of the bowel and anal continence. This operation is most successful when there is no perianal disease (significant anal fissures, hemorrhoids, or fistula) and may allow individuals to retain normal bowel function without severe diarrhea. In such cases, there is a significant chance of recurrence of the Crohn's disease, usually within the rectum, but in many instances the inflammation is insignificant and can be readily controlled with continued medical therapy. When such an option can be considered, most patients prefer to avoid an ileostomy and are willing to continue with medical treatment despite the potential inconvenience of more frequent bowel movements.

In patients who are unfortunate enough to have significant peri-anal Crohn's disease, one of the potential complications is the formation of abscesses around the anal canal or in the buttocks. When these abscesses become large or painful, they require an incision into the buttocks to allow the pus to drain out and may ultimately leave significant perianal scarring. One means of avoid-ing such a situation is for patients with perianal Crohn's disease to take meticulous care of this region with frequent sitz baths or by the use of a flexible hand-held shower head (or shower massage), which can be used to thoroughly cleanse the anal area, thereby washing away debris that can otherwise become caught in the creases of the buttocks and could form the locus of an infection or early abscess. Certain antibiotics such as metronidazole or tetracycline have also been found to be useful in many cases of significant perianal disease and can help control or prevent these local perianal complications. Unfortunately, certain individuals will continue to have recurrent problems that can only be controlled by diverting the fecal stream by the formation of an ileostomy or colostomy (Fig. 15). Usually this is the final stage of a long and frustrating course for both the patient and physician.

Sometimes the surgeon will find that a patient has gallstones at an operation for other indications in Crohn's disease. It may be advis-able under certain of these situations to remove the gallbladder so that future problems with gallstones can be avoided. A thorough evaluation prior to any surgery may identify such patients with ''silent'' gallstones so that the removal of the gallbladder can be planned prior to the actual operation. When this is not possible, the decision to remove a stone-filled gallbladder is at the discretion of the surgeon. Most patients will tolerate the operation without any significant problems, although a reduction in the amount of fatty or greasy foods may be helpful in adjusting to the removal of the gallbladder.

Another complication of Crohn's disease that at times requires surgery is the presence of kidney stones. Several newer, less in-vasive techniques for the surgical removal of kidney stones are becoming available, so that major operations that previously in-volved large incisions over the back are rarely necessary. Some

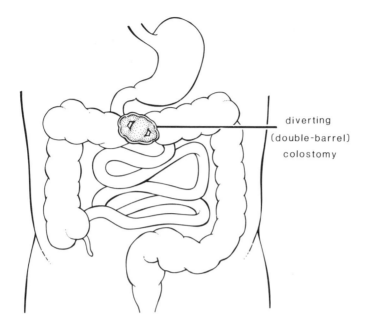

diverting
(double-barrel)
colostomy

FIG. 15. Diverting colostomy.

stones can be removed through the urinary bladder at cystoscopy, and others can be reached via a tube directed through the back, by the aid of an ultrasound machine, into the kidney. The stones then can be removed through this tube after additional ultrasonic "shock waves" break the larger stones into gravel. Eventually, it will be possible to aim the ultrasonic force at the kidneys without the use of any surgery so that these soundwaves will crush the stones, which can then pass through the urinary system and bladder. Once the stones have been analyzed, specific dietary measures may be helpful in avoiding recurrences.

After any surgery in Crohn's disease, it is important to continue follow-up visits to the primary care physician. It may be necessary to readjust or decrease medications as well as to manipulate an individual's diet for optimal results. After the immediate postoperative period, most individuals are able to resume a regular and vigorous life-style with few limitations. It is advisable to continue with medical check-ups at regular intervals so that changes in health or bowel habits can be reviewed when the problem is early and more readily dealt with. Often, increases in bowel movements are unrelated to active Crohn's disease and may be easily handled with dietary adjustments. On the other hand, since there is a substantial likelihood of a return of the inflammation, it is useful to recognize early symptoms of recurrent Crohn's disease so that medical therapy can be reinstituted and continuously controlled.

CHAPTER 11

Emotional Support

The spectrum of illness and complications of inflammatory bowel disease is wide, and the symptoms, restrictions on diet or activities, occasional visits to doctors, or hospitalizations may interfere with an individual's desired life-style. As with any chronic illness, the diagnosis of inflammatory bowel disease also can represent a major life crisis. Despite great improvements in our ability to manage these disorders, the symptoms, eventual diagnosis, and treatment impose a significant disruption of a (presumably) previously good adaptation to living for the patient. Often, the spouse, the parents, and the family bear a considerable brunt of the emotional consequences of the illness. At other times, the patient with inflammatory bowel disease becomes the focal point of an entire family's energies by virtue of intermittent flare-ups at home and periods in the hospital. Furthermore, an individual's occupation or schoolwork may suffer as a consequence, requiring the understanding and the flexibility of supervisors or teachers.

The family or the spouse must provide the first line of emotional support for the individual. In the case of children with inflammatory bowel disease, parents must allocate extraordinary energies to maintaining a harmonious balance between caring for the sick child and not emotionally abandoning other siblings. Great care must be taken that the ill child not receive the entire distribution of attention lest the other children become jealous of the malady. Also, such focusing of attention on a child's illness can actually be harmful if more attention is devoted to the disease than to maintaining the family

135

structure. When this occurs, the child may begin to identify more with being ill than with developing an interest in growing and maturing while adapting to a problem. To a minor degree, such arrests in development are inevitable when children become severely ill and/or are hospitalized; we strive to minimize these problems by being aware of them and by anticipating both the problem and, we hope, the solutions.

In the latter situation, the burden on the parents is tremendous, as they must share responsibilities in attending to their sick child while maintaining interest and concern for the rest of the family. The emotions of fear and guilt are often overwhelming to a young parent confronted with a child who becomes ill and is faced with the possibility of a chronic condition. If the family equilibrium is distorted sufficiently, the illness can insinuate itself between the parents and produce a schism that may require external professional assistance for support. This also is a time that can bring a husband and wife closer to each other emotionally.

When a spouse develops inflammatory bowel disease, the burdens can be equally severe. The new ailment produces an unanticipated change in the couple's expectations and life-style that, in the absence of a secure relationship, may be very divisive. It is easy to observe how intermittent sickness, hospitalization, and the possibility of disability or surgery can abruptly cancel a couple's plans for work, leisure, housing, or vacation. Even the consideration of raising a family may be altered in face of dealing with inflammatory bowel disease. The physician must be cognizant of the burdens related to the loss of income because of illness, increases in the expense of insurance and medical and surgical care, and loss of time and energy devoted to coping with an illness so that needed support can be anticipated and provided.

Despite the potential adversity, the strengths of family and husband–wife bonds typically rise to the occasion for the maintenance of the equilibrium needed to carry on as normal a family life as possible. A combination of understanding, sympathy, empathy, and, most of all, a strong, loving relationship are as important as any medications for the long-term well-being of the patient and his or her family. Certainly, ups and downs will be encountered, which greatly stress the family bonds. However, most family ties are more flexible than might be anticipated prior to a chronic illness, and the bonding cement will become even stronger by having withstood the crisis of a family member's illness.

Each individual and family can be expected to use an array of "coping mechanisms" in order to deal with the emotional stress of such an illness. The first reaction is typically denial of the true existence of a long-term problem. This may lead patients to minimize their symptoms, skip doses or discontinue medications, or, worse, ignore increasing problems until they are finally in dire straits prior to consulting their physician. Family denial may lead a parent to ignore the child's (husband's/wife's) complaints or consider them to be exaggerated or overemphasized. Although such an initial reaction may temporarily be injurious, the eventual response can be adaptive by protecting these individuals from becoming overwhelmed by feelings of catastrophe or guilt.

Periods of depression often follow. The individuals are, of course, saddened by their plight, but these emotions also represent a feeling of mourning over the "loss" of one's former self and ultimately are therapeutic once the individual moves forward.

During these intervals, issues of control often supervene. A patient may speak of a process that has "taken over" within his or her body, often feeling as if the disease is an external entity. This is a time when adolescents may rebel against authority figures (physicians or parents) and may further attempt to take their medical care into their own hands. A perceptive physician should recognize these issues and involve the patient in the decision-making processes leading to the therapeutic recommendations. When options are available, the patient should be encouraged to make his or her choices known. Here, the doctor(s) especially, but all of the involved staff (and relatives) can encourage the patient to strive for realistic independence yet to accept necessary areas of continued dependence.

At this point, as a patient you should be encouraged to speak up, to ask questions, and to negotiate actively for your demands. Ideally, the entire medical staff (physicians, nurses, aides, and ancillary personnel) will recognize your needs to understand and participate in the activities surrounding your care.

On the other hand, it is sometimes necessary to pace the "giving-out" of information. Deluging all patients with facts and details is not always the best approach initially, as each individual needs to assimilate the knowledge at his or her own rate and in a manner that allows him or her to retain control while not promoting undue obsessiveness. Such patterns tend to evolve related to issues of bowel function and may lead to overemphasis on personal activities or compulsive behavior.

The need to discuss bowel activity, a general taboo in our society, may also elicit feelings of embarrassment or shame unique to people with intestinal disorders. Furthermore, patients are expected to, literally, "expose" all parts of themselves for examinations in ways that a heart or lung problem does not require. The medical and support staff must respect and maintain "privacy" whenever possible.

An understanding and capable physician is essential in orchestrating medical and emotional care. Compassion from the doctor, an open relationship with the patient and his or her family, and most of all, the time to hear and sort out the patient's or family's turmoils in dealing with inflammatory bowel disease are requisites of a successful patient–physician relationship. In the absence of such a joint effort, patients and their families can struggle with feelings of fear, guilt, and uncertainty that can intensify the physical ailment.

The physician must also understand the vicissitudes of inflammatory bowel disease and be able to anticipate the questions, needs, and strains on an individual and the family. It is helpful if the doctor can be easily available (on virtually a 24-hour basis) for consultation regarding medical concerns, either major or insignificant, as experienced by the patient or relative. Ideally, the physician will also perceive where the strains are becoming overwhelming within a family unit and be able to provide the necessary insight and security to shore up or restructure the instabilities. Often, it is not the physician alone who provides such back-up support. It may be a nurse within the office setting or even a compassionate secretary or office-worker who is familiar with the patient and family and can sense when more emotional support is necessary. Often such crises revolve around missing items of information or fears of the unknown that can be easily calmed. At times, an individual may not want to reveal his or her concerns to the physician, yet may be more willing to "talk" to one of the nursing or technical associates. Whoever the medical person is who is confronted with the problem, open lines of communication within the medical team are important in subduing a smoldering fire or spark before the issue is out of control.

The hospital environment is frequently helpful from the standpoint of enhanced emotional support. Here, more nurses are available in a nurturing role, medical students and/or house officers review in detail the patient's medical and personal history, and in many units, social workers and/or psychiatric consultants are available to handle more severe problems. In the ideal therapeutic milieu, such support comes from many directions. Having several patients with similar problems in the hospital at the same time can be most comforting and reassuring for individuals who can then see that they are not isolated by rare conditions. At times, close relationships with fellow patients may become frightening if complications occur or if things do not always go as anticipated, and the hospital staff should be prepared to intervene with explanations to observers. The staff should also emphasize the differences between individual "cases" so that patients and families understand that "what is happening" to others need not apply to themselves. In any event, observing another individual or family coping with similar problems will usually be beneficial and may be the catalyst for rallying one's own coping mechanisms and security.

One question that is frequently posed is whether "stress" plays a role in inflammatory bowel disease. Most patients recognize that "stress" aggravates their medical condition. In reality, this is not limited to inflammatory bowel disease, as, for example, life stresses can intensify coronary artery disease leading to heart attacks or make a diabetic's control of blood sugar worse. However, because inflammatory bowel disease was once labeled a psychiatric or psychosomatic condition, individuals are often concerned that their condition represents an inadequate coping mechanism for stressful situations. A corollary question is then "Should I see a therapist?"

We do not recommend psychologic or psychiatric support for the majority of our patients. However, we do tend to use a very supportive environment both in the outpatient setting and within the hospital, and we attempt to generate additional support from the individual family members as mentioned in the preceding paragraphs. However, in certain instances it is reasonable to incorporate a psychotherapist into our environment for patients who are having an unusually difficult time coping with the inflammatory bowel disease for whatever reason. Again, we must emphasize that the majority of our patients are capable of dealing with much adversity, considering the degree of physical and emotional turmoil that they, at times, may confront. Recent studies that have reexamined the question of underlying psychologic problems in patients with inflammatory bowel disease have, for the most part, not identified any consistent underlying problems with patients before they develop inflammatory bowel disease. As one might expect, feelings of depression may develop with inflammatory bowel disease, but these do not seem to be prominent before the onset of symptoms.

As would be found in any group of individuals, a number of patients will have more than the average difficulty in adjusting to the medical and emotional problems of inflammatory bowel disease. For these individuals, psychologic counseling may be most useful. We do not expect that psychotherapy will completely change an individual's personality structure so that he or she can ''cure'' his or her inflammatory condition; yet, various forms of psychiatric counseling may help an individual by teaching methods of handling the additional emotional burden of his or her illness. A variety of techniques may be useful, ranging from intensive psychotherapy to biofeedback or even meditation. No one technique is right for every individual, and some expertise must be utilized in consulting the appropriate therapist for each patient.

The psychologic consultant must be familiar with patients with inflammatory bowel disease as well as the effects of medications that are used (most importantly steroids). Cortisone and its derivatives can exaggerate normal emotional swings at both extremes. We see many individuals who become quite elated while on cortisone, whereas others can become severely depressed. Most patients have a mixture of the two and notice their own mood swings, which are just slightly exaggerated. At times, steroids may unmask a previously unnoticed underlying depression or personality disorder, in which case the response can be quite severe. In these circumstances, medications to counteract the severe depression may be warranted, especially in the rare circumstance where suicide is threatened. Such a situation would call for intensive psychiatric support and observation, usually within the hospital.

In most circumstances, however, stronger medications than the low doses of sedatives that are frequently used for symptoms of abdominal pain will not be necessary. Again, the physician must be aware that some medications used for pain and sedation (such as barbiturates) can also act as depressants. Naturally, if a patient seems to be swinging towards depression, caution must be exercised to avoid potentially complicating medications, and we often recommend a total review of all the medicines that are being taken to be sure that we are not dealing with a drug-related phenomenon. Nevertheless, there will be times when antianxiety or antidepressant medications may be useful in the overall therapeutic setting, at which time direct communication among all of the consulting physicians and the patient will insure that the appropriate medication will be used.

Sometimes the emotional impact of inflammatory bowel disease will fall harder on another family member rather than on the patient. For instance, parents can be overwhelmed with guilt or sadness related to a sick child; a spouse may have difficulty accepting the physical restrictions on his or her mate; or a sibling rivalry may be intensified by the attention given to the sick brother or sister with resultant jealousy. Such events are not at all unusual and are often aided by family counseling with a therapist (psychologist, psychiatrist, or social worker). Such meetings can solidify family bonds and equalize or distribute pressures among family members rather than focusing all of the good and/or bad energy on a single individual.

OTHER SUPPORT ORGANIZATIONS

Outside the medical system, organizations have been formed by individuals with similar problems and needs to provide additional support, patient education, and research funding. One such organization has been created specifically related to inflammatory bowel disease and now has chapters nationwide. The National Foundation for Ileitis and Colitis (National Headquarters, 444 Park Avenue South, 11th Floor, New York, NY 10016) is oriented toward patient and family support, educational teaching, and conferences for patients with inflammatory bowel disease; it functions in a fund-raising capacity as well to generate research money for all aspects of inflammatory bowel disease. Interested parties may participate in whatever manner they desire, as members of a patient/family work group or as counselors, and/or involve themselves with a variety of the many realms within a national organization committed to improving the plight of patients with inflammatory bowel disease.

Other groups have formed revolving around the use of ostomies. The Ileoptimists, Ostomates, and local Ileostomy Foundations are examples of groups that have formed for mutual support and information relating to the special needs of these individuals. The United Ostomy Association is a national organization that may direct patients to smaller working groups and may, as well, be able to provide discounts and information related to ostomy supplies. Names of local chapters can often be obtained from the enterostomal nurses at nearby hospitals (see also Appendix to Chapter 13).

One can often turn to church groups, community networks, or, at times, even corporation-related groups for counseling. Patients and their families should consult their physician, nurse, or social worker when they recognize needs that are not being met by the medical system.

Local governmental agencies also may be a source of assistance. For instance, if an individual should lose his or her job or medical insurance, the services of a local Human Service Organization (city or state), or the Social Security Office (federal) may be employed. At times it may be necessary to apply for public assistance (state public aid) to meet medical expenses when all other resources have been exhausted.

A corollary to this discussion is the suggestion that a patient with inflammatory bowel disease should *never* allow his or her current medical insurance policy to lapse. Although physicians and organizations such as the NFIC are working in concert to improve the insurability of patients, most insurance companies will *not* insure patients with preexisting ulcerative colitis or Crohn's disease. Individual policies are virtually impossible to obtain, although many larger group policies will be able to incorporate patients with existing chronic ailments. When confronted with such a situation, it may be helpful to obtain a written statement from one's physician documenting the status of the illness to support one's application. Unfortunately, the above consideration may also apply to patients (or spouses) who are contemplating job changes, in which case they should explore their present insurance, the potential transferability (if any) and interim coverage, and the new company's policy prior to making a final decision.

When one's occupation has been temporarily interrupted, the Department of Rehabilitation Services (in some states) may be utilized, or the Social Security Office may provide disability income in appropriate situations. Finally, when disputes over matters of insurance, medical expenses, loss of jobs, etc. develop, either the Legal Aid Bureau, Legal Assistance Foundation, American Civil Liberties Union, or state Department of Insurance may be consulted.

CHAPTER 12

Inflammatory Bowel Disease in Children

BARBARA S. KIRSCHNER

Many people tend to think of Crohn's disease and ulcerative colitis as disorders of adulthood, yet studies from several centers have shown that at least 20% of patients have signs of these conditions before 20 years of age. The majority of these children are diagnosed between 10 and 18 years and, rarely, before 4 years, with boys and girls equally affected. Ulcerative colitis used to be diagnosed more often than Crohn's disease in children. However, there appears to be a leveling of the increase in new cases of ulcerative colitis (incidence), whereas Crohn's disease continues to be on the increase and pediatric patients are now more likely to have Crohn's disease than ulcerative colitis. The majority (75%) of children and adolescents do not have a family history of either of these conditions. Therefore, when the diagnosis is confirmed , it is often the family's first awareness that these conditions exist. This chapter discusses some of the aspects of inflammatory bowel disease that are particular to children and adolescents.

SYMPTOMS OF INFLAMMATORY BOWEL DISEASE IN CHILDREN

Abdominal pain is the most frequent symptom described by children with inflammatory bowel disease. At first, the discomfort may be infrequent and of short duration. As the inflammation progresses in untreated patients, the pain increases in intensity, frequency, and duration. The nature and location of the pain may be clues to the region of the intestine that is inflamed. Crohn's disease of the small intestine seems to provoke feelings of cramping in association with or soon after eating. The discomfort usually is felt around the umbilicus (navel, "belly button") or in the right lower portion of the abdomen and results from food being propelled through the inflamed, narrowed segment of bowel following a meal. Physicians refer to this as the gastrocolic reflex. Crohn's disease of the colon and ulcerative colitis usually are associated with cramping pain that occurs just before and is relieved by bowel movements. The pain in these situations usually is more diffuse and is felt across the lower abdomen.

It should be emphasized that at times the pain may be perceived by the child (or patient) as so mild and infrequent that it is not thought to reflect a real illness. Often, the early complaints are ascribed to problems related to schoolwork, "laziness," or difficulties in social adjustments. In a few childen, pain is not a prominent feature, thus delaying the time that medical attention is sought.

Most children and adolescents will notice a *change in their stool pattern*. Usually, the number of daily stools will increase with a looser consistency. If pain is prominent, however, the decrease in appetite may actually lead to constipation in 20% of pediatric patients. The latter is especially true if the disease is initially limited to the terminal ileum. At times, an adolescent's strong sense of privacy delays informing his or her parents of these experiences until they occur repeatedly. The appearance of blood is usually sufficient for them to seek parental and medical advice sooner. Although obvious bleeding may occur in Crohn's disease of the small bowel, it is much more likely to represent ulcerative colitis or Crohn's disease of the colon. Hence, the presence of blood often results in ulcerative colitis being diagnosed within weeks after the onset of symptoms. In contrast, the diagnosis of Crohn's disease may be delayed for months or even years.

Weight loss or *failure to gain weight* at the expected rate is a very significant feature of childhood inflammatory bowel disease. We have observed that 87% of children with Crohn's disease have lost weight (averaging 12.5 lb) at the time of diagnosis. This was less frequent (67%) and of lesser degree (9.1 lb) in ulcerative colitis, most likely reflecting a more rapid diagnosis after the onset of symptoms. The cause of the weight loss is the gradual diminution in food intake as the child attempts (often unconsciously) to lessen the intensity and frequency of the gastrointestinal symptoms. This aspect is discussed more fully later in this chapter.

Recognized *fever* may be noted in almost half of pediatric patients. Chills or night sweats may be subtle manifestations of undocumented fevers, which are present when the inflammatory process is active, that is, in untreated patients during acute flare-up of the condition. The disappearance of these symptoms may be useful signs of the effectiveness of medical treatment.

Joint pain is a frequent complaint, occurring in approximately one-quarter of children with inflammatory bowel disease. Usually, there is discomfort (arthralgia) without actual swelling or redness of the joint (arthritis). The large joints, especially the ankles, knees, and wrists, are most often affected. The pain typically occurs during a period when there is active intestinal inflammation, although, as with adults, this is not always the case. Conversely, the pain usually subsides with treatment of the underlying bowel disease. Specific antiinflammatory medications may be cautiously prescribed (remembering these drugs' capacity to cause stomach irritation) to relieve persistent or severe joint pain. Fortunately, in contrast to other forms of juvenile arthritis, deformity of the joints does not occur in inflammatory bowel disease. The only exception is the presence of a rare form of arthritis of the spine, ankylosing spondylitis, which does cause progressive stiffness of the lower spine.

Clubbing (rounding) of the fingers also occurs in up to 25% of children with Crohn's disease, most prominently with extensive small bowel disease. It may improve or disappear following remission of disease activity in the intestines.

Lesions of the mucus membranes (gums and mouth) called aphthous ulcers are not unusual in children with inflammatory bowel disease. As with the other extraintestinal symptoms, they are common in untreated patients or during an acute flare–up of disease activity. Skin lesions may appear in two main forms—flat lesions with a dark or ulcerated center or raised red or purple nodules (erythema nodosum). They are thought to represent involvement of small blood vessels in the skin and, again, usually correspond to activity of the intestinal disease, with resolution coinciding with satisfactory response of the bowel disease to medical management. Special medications and methods of skin care will, on occasion, be necessary.

Growth failure is an important complication of childhood inflammatory bowel disease. We have observed that over one-third of children and adolescents with Crohn's disease have developed an abnormal slowing of the growth rate by the time the condition is first diagnosed. This is less likely to occur in ulcerative colitis (14% of children) since, as mentioned earlier, this condition tends to be diagnosed sooner. At times, the impaired growth occurs before any gastrointestinal or other disease is recognized.

In order to determine whether growth has been affected, the doctor must plot the child's height on standard height curves. It is very useful to have such information from earlier childhood so that the physician can compare the height percentile (a comparison of height for age) to see if there is a change. If this is not available, we can estimate that a child or teenager should grow approximately 2 inches per year until sexual maturation is complete. Rates lower than this need to be evaluated by physicians with experience in analyzing growth problems.

Noting that the child is lower than average on the growth chart does not in itself indicate that he or she has growth failure. Some children are short because of a familial pattern (genetic short stature). Others have a form of normal delay in growth that will improve with age (constitutional delayed growth). If there is a suspicion of impaired growth, the physician needs to review growth data and determine the skeletal age with appropriate X-rays of the bones in hand. These will allow the doctor to predict how much additional growth potential remains.

Investigations in several centers have shown that levels of growth hormone (a chemical messenger that induces growth) are normal in children with inflammatory bowel disease. In fact, some studies have reported that levels may actually be higher than in children without inflammatory bowel disease. In one very small test group, injections of growth hormone did not promote improved growth in any child with inflammatory bowel disease. These findings have suggested that other hormones (such as somatomedin) may have a role in the retardation of growth in inflammatory bowel disease, and research is under way to evaluate how these hormones influence the growth rate in affected children.

It might seem that the weight loss and poor growth could be caused by an inability of the inflamed intestine to absorb nutrients normally. This does not seem to be true in most instances, as studies have demonstrated sufficient intestinal absorptive capacity in most affected children. Hence, it is currently thought that diminished intake of nutrients is the most significant factor explaining the reduced growth rate. We have shown that children with abnormal growth consume, on the average, only 50% of the recommended calories for children their age. Increasing the calorie intake to at least 90% of that recommended for age was usually sufficient to reverse the growth arrest (induce a growth spurt). This improved nutritional state can result from enhanced oral intake of food (with or without special supplemental formulas) or from intravenous (parenteral) nutrition. The details of therapy for this problem are discussed later.

It is important that children and adolescents with inflammatory bowel disease have their growth carefully checked at 3- to 6-month intervals. If growth has been severely affected, it may require 3 or 4 years of medical treatment and control of the disease for the original height percentile to be achieved. In the setting of continuous disease activity, the final adult stature may be less than predicted from estimates of potential achievable height.

When inflammatory bowel disease affects children prior to the onset of puberty, the subsequent development of secondary sexual characteristics (breast development, beard, pubic hair, etc.) of these patients may be significantly delayed. In most instances, control of the disease activity and improved nutritional status will then allow pubertal development to proceed normally. However, active disease frequently influences the regularity of menstrual periods in girls. In fact, weight loss or significant illness is often associated with a temporary cessation of menses, which return when there is satisfactory weight gain.

LABORATORY TESTS

Many of the diagnostic studies that have been described earlier in this book also apply to children. To some degree, the frequency with which procedures are performed may be lessened because of their potential emotional affect on children. However, it is important that pediatric patients and their parents recognize that looking directly at the intestinal lining (proctoscopy or colonoscopy) is a very important method for determining the degree of disease activity, which will then allow the physician to plan and adjust the medical therapy.

X-Ray studies provide further details regarding the extent and severity of the intestinal inflammation. Although physicians should attempt to limit repeated X-ray studies in children, at times they are necessary to determine whether a significant change has taken place and whether therapy should be altered in a major way.

Blood tests usually include a blood count to exclude anemia, an erythrocyte sedimentation rate (ESR), which often reflects disease activity, serum proteins, and selected mineral and vitamin levels. If abnormalities are found, the test may need to be repeated until the values have improved.

MEDICAL MANAGEMENT

Medications used in the treatment of children and adolescents with inflammatory bowel disease need to be considered from the viewpoint of the growing patient. Therefore, there is sometimes hesitation to use certain medications in children that are known to be helpful in adults because of their special consequences for children.

Sulfasalazine (Azulfidine®) is widely used in pediatric patients with both ulcerative colitis and Crohn's disease. As with adults, mild to moderate side effects are common. By beginning with a low dose and gradually increasing the amount over several days, headaches are encountered less frequently. A similar schedule may avoid gastrointestinal discomfort, which may also be alleviated by taking the drug with meals. Still, there are some children who develop a rash or other allergic symptoms that may necessitate a change to another medication.

Corticosteroid medications (prednisone, methylprednisolone, Medrol®, hydrocortisone) are the most effective medications used to control active intestinal inflammation. Depending on the severity of the symptoms, they are given by mouth or intravenously. In general, these preparations are given on a daily basis for at least 4 to 6 weeks in an attempt to decrease intestinal inflammation and the child's symptoms. When there are signs of disease control, the physician attempts to gradually change (taper) the corticosteroids to an alternate-day (every-other-day) schedule. The major value of this approach is that it may control symptoms and at the same time permit the child to grow at a normal rate. The unpleasant cosmetic side effects of corticosteroids (including facial roundness, weight gain, hair growth, and acne) decrease significantly with every-other-day treatment. If symptoms do not subside, then other medications may be added to permit a lowering of the daily dose of corticosteroids.

Metronidazole (Flagyl®) has been shown to be effective in certain adult patients with Crohn's disease. Potential side effects include a metallic taste or nausea, an occasional "coated" tongue, and a rarely encountered but significant numbness or paresthesia (tingling) in the hands or feet. Although the long-term safety of this drug in children is not known, it is successful in controlling disease activity in some cases.

Azathioprine (Imuran®) and 6-mercaptopurine (6-MP) are immune system suppressant drugs that are reported to be useful in adult patients with inflammatory bowel disease, particularly Crohn's disease. Again, long-term safety of these preparations in children is not known. However, pediatric gastroenterologists in several centers have successfully used these preparations in a select few patients in an attempt to control symptoms and decrease daily prednisone requirements.

A severe increase in activity of the intestinal inflammation or the occurrence of significant complications will, at times, have a better

chance of resolving if the bowel is rested from the work of digestion. The administration of sufficient fluids by vein to meet the
body's requirements may preempt the need for nutrition by mouth
and permit the bowel to rest. These measures may be suggested in
the presence of moderate or severe pain or diarrhea, peristent or
recurrent fever, an abdominal mass, intestinal obstruction, excessive bleeding, suspected infection, fissures, or fistulas. The period of time that the intravenous fluids are used will depend on the
speed and completeness of the response to the overall medical program.

NUTRITIONAL INTERVENTION

As has been continuously emphasized, the nutritional state of the
patient (especially children and teenagers) is vitally important in
achieving a positive course of the inflammatory bowel disease.
Some clinicians have observed that nutritionally depleted patients
do not appear to respond well to medications, particularly to corticosteroids. The impairment of growth (height), poor weight gain,
and delayed sexual maturation have been clearly related, at least in
part, to an inadequate caloric intake. In addition, specific mineral
(for example, iron) and vitamin deficiencies (folic acid, vitamins A,
D, B_{12}) result from a combination of altered dietary consumption,
medication affects, and impaired intestinal absorption. The
approach to improving the nutritional status varies according to the
severity of the undernutrition as well as the child's ability to tolerate
food.

The initial steps towards improving the nutritional status of the
child are first to assess the degree of undernutrition and then to
establish caloric and protein goals that are appropriate for the child's
height, age, and sex. Nutritionists, dieticians, and physicians may
consult special tables (recommended dietary allowances), which are
available for this purpose. In general, for patients in the 12- to
16-year range, approximately 2,400 to 3,000 calories and 50 to 60
grams of protein are necessary for most patients. Clearly, the gastrointestinal symptoms must be controlled before children are able
to attain these goals, which will enable them to resume their normal
daily activity and to grow normally.

When possible, improvement in nutritional status is attempted using dietary changes, sometimes with special supplemental liquid formulas. This is an area in which specific recommmendations may vary between physicians. In general, if the bowel is narrowed from inflammation (as one sees with Crohn's disease), cramping symptoms are often decreased by foods that are physically soft and low in unabsorbable fiber. Raw fruits and vegetables, nuts, seeds, and whole-grain breads usually are temporarily excluded on this diet. A similar regimen may be recommended for patients with excessive diarrhea in an attempt to decrease the amount of stool production.

In some children, milk or milk products may cause abdominal distention or bloating, gaseousness, cramping, or diarrhea. These patients should be evaluated for lactase deficiency. Lactase is an intestinal enzyme that digests milk sugar (lactose). If the sugar is incompletely digested and is partially absorbed, the symptoms described above may occur. Since milk may be an important source of calories, protein, and calcium in childhood, the tolerance of milk should be determined if symptoms occur. There are two methods for measuring lactose malabsorption—a hydrogen breath test and a blood test to assess absorption. There are currently commercial products available (LactAid®, Lactrase™) can be added to milk to digest the milk sugar before it is consumed. This enables the lactose-intolerant child to continue to drink milk if desired.

In order to achieve the goals described above, it is often necessary for the child or adolescent to discuss food preferences with a dietician or nutritionist. If this approach is not sufficient to provide adequate calories from regular foods, then additional calories (and nutrients) can be added by liquid formulas. There are many preparations available, so that a child will be able to select his or her preference, which allows an overall better acceptance by these "choosy" eaters.

At times, dietary intake remains inadequate despite the above-mentioned approaches. Some investigators have shown that infusing nutrients through a soft tube placed through the nose and swallowed into the stomach during sleep can be effective in improving weight gain and growth. The nasogastric tube is then removed in the morning before the child goes to school. At times, this same method is used in hospitalized patients to achieve disease control and weight gain. If the desired increase in weight cannot be achieved using enteral (intestinal) methods, then intravenous nutritional support may be necessary.

In recent years, it has become possible to supply the total nutritional requirements intravenously for extended periods of time. The procedure may be performed using peripheral veins (in the arm) or central veins (large veins near the heart). The latter are reached by minor surgical procedures to place the catheter under the clavical (collar bone) into the subclavian vein or into the lower neck above the clavicle into the jugular vein. When all of the nutrition is supplied intravenously, the process is termed hyperalimentation or total parenteral nutrition (TPN). Although the use of peripheral veins requires hospitalization, patients with central venous catheters can be taught to administer their fluids at home following a period of training in the hospital. The potential complications and enormous cost of TPN make the selection of appropriate patients critical for successful outcome. Furthermore, TPN should probably be reserved for patients in whom at least 2 weeks of intravenous support is required.

Nevertheless, this important advancement is therapy has greatly affected the management of pediatric inflammatory bowel disease. It is, at times, indicated in the following circumstances: (a) providing bowel rest to decrease severe gastrointestinal symptoms (pain, diarrhea, inflammatory mass, fistula), (b) repleting an undernourished patient who cannot be improved by the intestinal route, (c) preparing a malnourished patient for surgery, (d) providing ongoing nutritional support for patients with extensive small bowel disease or a ''short bowel'' after multiple or lengthy intestinal resections, (e) promoting growth in some severely growth-impaired children who do not respond to oral methods.

SURGERY IN CHILDHOOD INFLAMMATORY BOWEL DISEASE

Ulcerative Colitis

At least 25% of pediatric patients with ulcerative colitis undergo surgical resection of the colon. The frequency is greatest in those children with early onset and extensive colonic involvement (pancolitis). In some instances, the duration of the symptoms may be only a few weeks, whereas in others, the activity may have "flared up" following a remission or have remained poorly controlled over long intervals.

The usual reasons for surgery in childhood are: (a) excessive bleeding (hemorrhage), (b) acute dilatation of the colon (toxic megacolon), (c) poor response to medical management, and (d) growth failure in spite of good medical management.

Precancerous pathologic changes (dysplasia) in the intestinal lining cells also may be an indication for recommending colectomy. The risk of developing a precancer or a true malignancy increases with the length of time that ulcerative colitis has been present. For this reason, life-long surveillance is absolutely necessary for all pediatric patients with ulcerative colitis, and for this reason, it is our practice that teenagers who have had ulcerative colitis for more than 7 years have a colonoscopic examination with multiple biopsies at 1- to 2-year intervals to determine whether dysplasia is present.

If surgery is performed, several procedures are currently available (see Chapter 10). To some degree, the selection may be influenced by the urgency of the medical situation and the experience of the surgeon. Suffice it to say that the new ileoanal procedure (which uses the rectum for defecation rather than an external appliance) is currently undergoing a reevaluation and resurgence in the pediatric surgeon's approach to the treatment of ulcerative colitis.

Crohn's Disease

Whereas it was once thought that removal of the inflamed intestine along with the adjacent normal tissue would prevent the recurrence of Crohn's disease, unfortunately, this has not been shown to be true. In fact, the risk of a recurrence of Crohn's disease after surgery is approximately 40% at 5 years and increases to 90% at 15 years. Therefore, surgery is not able to "cure" Crohn's disease, and, for this reason, the decision regarding when to operate is usually made in the presence of complications rather than strictly for "active disease."

In some situations, surgery is usually necessary: (a) intestinal obstruction that does not respond to medical management, (b) suspected abdominal abscess, (c) persistent pain or symptoms that interfere with reasonable life-style (particularly when the area of involvement is limited), (d) growth retardation in a prepubertal or early pubertal patient who is not responding to medical management, or (e) extension to involve the urinary tract either by pressure on a ureter or fistula into the bladder.

Whenever possible, the area of direct involvement is removed (resected), and normal appearing bowel on each side is then connected together. If there is infection in the abdomen or in other rare situations, a temporary ileostomy may be necessary, which may then be closed following a period of recuperation. If the entire colon needs to be resected, the ileostomy is permanent. The new ileoanal procedure is rarely performed for Crohn's disease because of the risk of recurrence.

When an ileostomy is needed in a child, and particularly in adolescents, it can be enormously helpful to arrange for someone with an ileostomy of similar age and sex to meet with the child. Seeing how well these patients have adapted to the procedure can give encouragement to the youngster facing this situation. The same advice may also be appreciated by children and adolescents anticipating an intestinal resection or ileoanal anastomosis.

EMOTIONAL IMPACT OF INFLAMMATORY BOWEL DISEASE IN CHILDREN AND ADOLESCENTS

It is clear to all that for the patient and family, a period of adjustment is to be expected once a diagnosis of inflammatory bowel disease has been established. Furthermore, the problems of younger children are likely to be somewhat different from those of adolescents. For young children, the fear of examinations and even moderately invasive procedures (e.g., blood drawing, i.v.s, proctoscopic examinations) has the potential of adversely affecting the otherwise trusting relationship that should develop between patient and physician. Therefore, a compromise situation may exist for a while in which certain examinations may not be performed as often as the physician might wish, and for the more intrusive procedures the use of sedation can be very important to lower the level of anxiety and discomfort. Visiting hours should be liberalized in appropriate situations for parents of hospitalized children (including rooming-in) to lessen the fear of separation.

On the other hand, the attention to stool pattern invites or prolongs an involvement of parents in what would normally become an independent function for the child. There is sometimes a tendency for parents to continue their direct observations of this function longer than is appropriate for the child, and it may more appropriately be monitored by the nursing staff. Other duties, such as the distribution and taking of medications on a regular basis, may be shared and eventually transferred to the ultimately responsible individual. Such structure can even be worked into the child's learning schedule (e.g., dosages and mathematics) and responsibilities of maturation.

Adolescents, not unexpectedly, face some very different problems. At a time of intense peer pressure and conformity, they often resent having a condition that sets them apart. For this reason, and in attempting to prove their own independence, teenagers may take medications irregularly or discontinue their use. If the condition has been relatively quiet, it may take a few weeks or months for the activity to flare up again. The intervening interval may provide a false sense of reassurance, and denial that the subsequent flare-up is at all related to the stopping of the medications may supervene. This tendency can be diminished or thwarted by informing the teenage patients with ulcerative colitis that relapses are known to occur in only 20% of patients who continue sulfasalazine but in 80% of patients who do not take their medications. This further supports the teenage patient's own independence and decision making. Unfortunately, similar assurance is not available with regard to the risk of relapse in Crohn's disease.

In both age groups, anger or depression may accompany the reactivation of the intestinal disease. Both responses may be related to disappointment and recognition that the disorder has not been cured. Parents and physician should acknowledge this frustration and reiterate with optimism that management is possible and that all should work together to improve the inflammatory process as quickly as is possible. At times, professional counseling may help adolescents (and/or their families) cope with the anticipated fluctuations in the course of these diseases. The opportunity to meet and talk with other teenagers with these conditions, either alone or in a structured support group, lessens the isolation that some patients feel.

There is sometimes a tendency for parents to become overly protective of children and adolescents with inflammatory bowel disease. In general, teenagers should participate in all activities to the extent that they can. In some patients, certain gymnastic activities (particularly running) may exacerbate symptoms. If that occurs, a modified gym program may be necessary for a period. At all times, common sense should prevail, and the patients should "listen to their bodies" and reduce their activities in response to worsening symptoms.

Another potential source of school conflict concerns bathroom privileges. Even young children might wish privacy with regard to functions of elimination. It is often necessary for parents to arrange with teachers that children and adolescents may leave the classroom as needed in an independent manner without drawing attention to themselves. Furthermore, if the lavatories do not have doors, permission to use special facilities (such as the teacher's room) may have to be obtained.

It may be necessary to supply students with pamphlets in order to inform their teachers and principals about inflammatory bowel disease. This additional information may negate any outmoded concepts attributing inflammatory bowel disease to nervous or psychomatic causes. Ultimately, a conference between school authorities and the parents, with input from the physician, may prove to be of benefit.

CONCLUSIONS

Although the course of ulcerative colitis or Crohn's disease cannot be predicted in an individual case, pediatric patients function well most of the time. The medical approaches are usually successful in suppressing intestinal inflammation enough to permit a resumption of normal activity. At times, symptoms may be protracted, and hospitalization may be required, resulting in disappointment, anger, or depression. The support of parents and teachers and the interest of friends are critically important during these intervals; an experienced, understanding physician should communicate with both the patient and parents to anticipate and alleviate their stated and unstated fears. Eventually, learning to cope with these conditions permits the child to acknowledge the presence of these disorders while allowing him or her to concentrate on more productive areas in his or her life.

CHAPTER 13

Life with an Ostomy

JANICE C. COLWELL

Over 100,000 people in the United States and Canada have abdominal stomas. Despite this large number of individuals, few people are fully informed about the nature of stomas and their management. Those individuals who have heard of a colostomy or ileostomy have only a vague idea of stomas and their care. This chapter explains the nature of stomas and the adjustments necessary to living with a stoma.

Stoma and ostomy are derived from the Latin meaning mouth or opening. There are three common abdominal stomas: ileostomy (opening into the ileum), colostomy (opening into the colon), and urostomy (opening into the urinary system). These surgically created stomas discharge waste material, which is collected by an appliance or pouch attached to the skin around the stoma. The following discussion is limited to ileostomies and colostomies.

ILEOSTOMY

The small intestine is divided into three sections: the duodenum, the jejunum, and the ileum. An ileostomy is a surgically created opening into the terminal or end portion of the ileum. In order to preserve the digestive and absorptive functions, the entirety of the small intestine is kept intact though disconnected from the colon,

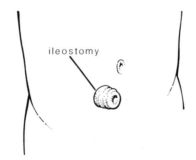

FIG. 16. Ileostomy.

and the end of the ileum is brought out through an opening in the skin. This surgically created opening discharges the end product of digestion, in a liquid form, into an externally worn appliance or bag. The function of the colon is to absorb fluid from the stool and to store the stool as it passes out of the body via the rectum. Because an ileostomy diverts the stool away from the colon, the stool has a liquid to pasty consistency and passes out of the ileostomy several times a day.

The ileostomy stoma (or opening) is usually located on the lower right quadrant of the abdomen. The surgeon creates an opening in the abdominal wall and brings the end of the ileum out through this opening. The surface lining (mucosa) is inverted (folded over on itself) and sewn onto the skin (see Fig. 16).

The location of the ileostomy stoma is very important. Prior to the operation, the site is determined jointly by the surgeon and the enterostomal nurse therapist (nurse specializing in stoma care). The abdomen is viewed in the sitting and lying position. Skin folds and creases are noted, old scars are identified, and the position of the belt line is noted. Ideally, the spot where the ileostomy is placed should have a 2-inch circular area free of creases, folds, or scars and lie below the level of the belt line. It is also important that the patient be able to view the stoma easily to facilitate its care. Proper placement will provide flexibility of movement and will not disturb the seal of the appliance. The spot is then marked with indelible ink prior to surgery.

The ileostomy stoma should eventually protrude ¾ to 1 inch above the skin surface. This allows the stool to be discharged directly into the appliance. The stoma diameter varies from person to person but generally is 1 to 2 inches around.

The lining of the small intestine is similar to the lining inside the mouth; hence, the stoma "skin" is red, moist, and shiny. It always remains so, since skin will not grow around it.

There are no pain receptors (nerves) in the stoma. Therefore, the stoma feels no pain when touched; there is no sensation of stool passage. For this reason, an appliance or pouch must be worn at all times. The appliance collects the residual bowel content until it is convenient to collect and dispose of it.

Care of Ileostomy

Skin Care

The stool from the ileostomy contains gastric juices and enzymes that could cause damage if they come in contact with the skin. As a result, the peristomal skin (area around the stoma) must be protected at all times. A skin barrier is a product that covers the peristomal skin and provides protection against the stool when the stoma drains. The appropriate skin barrier is based on the size of the stoma and the condition of the surrounding skin. A very common product is a 4 × 4 inch gelatinous wafer with adhesive on one side. An opening the same size as the stoma is cut from the wafer. The adhesive side is placed against the peristomal skin, fitting flush up to the stoma (see Fig. 17). The skin barrier usually will remain in place 3 to 5 days and needs to be changed when it begins to melt down. The melting down process depends on the type and amount of stool that comes in contact with the wafer. High volumes of ileostomy output, because of their enzyme content, often cause the skin barrier to melt down faster.

Several companies manufacture skin barriers (see Appendix). The ideal product stays in place for 5 days and is flexible enough to move with the wearer.

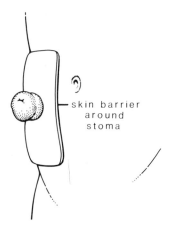

skin barrier
around
stoma

FIG. 17. Stoma with skin barrier.

Appliances

The average output from an ileostomy is approximately 1 to 1½ quarts over 24 hours. The ileostomy appliance (bag/pouch) can be drained, allowing the contents to be emptied as necessary without removal from the body. Removing the appliance several times a day would damage the adjacent skin.

The ileostomy appliance must meet three criteria. It should (a) maintain a seal against the body for 4 to 5 days, (b) allow the stool to be drained as necessary, and (c) contain no odor. Several companies manufacture pouches. The one chosen depends on the size and location of the stoma and the wearer's preference.

An average ileostomy appliance is approximately 10 to 12 inches in length with adhesive around the stoma opening (see Fig. 18). The adhesive patch attaches to the skin barrier and holds the pouch on the body. The pouches are available in various shapes and materials. Generally, a clear 12 inch appliance is used immediately after surgery to allow visualization of the stoma and stool. An opaque or patterned pouch is then used after the patient is discharged from the hospital.

The appliance opening (the part that fits around the stoma) should approximate the size of the stoma. Pouches come presized or with no opening, allowing the user more flexibility in adjusting the hole size. Presized pouches generally begin with a 1-inch opening and increase by ¼-inch increments to 3-inch openings.

Ileostomy pouches are available in either disposable or reusable styles. Disposable pouches can be worn for 3 to 5 days, removed, and discarded. They are drained several times a day by removing a clamp at the bottom, emptying the contents, and replacing the clamp. They are constructed of lightweight plastic and come in different shapes and in various colors (opaque, beige, blue, etc.).

Reusable appliances, as the name implies, can be reused. The faceplate is composed of a round or oval disk that is custom fit to the stoma and peristomal area. The faceplate is made of rubber or plastic and is available in various convexities and in different degrees of firmness for individual comfort. The drainable pouch connects to the faceplate by fitting over a small collar and attaches to the skin by use of a double-faced adhesive disk (see Fig. 19). The faceplate is fit ⅛ inch larger than the stoma to accomodate enlargement of the stoma as stool passes out. The peristomal skin is protected with a washer of any of the available skin barriers. The system then stays in place for 4 to 7 days. The pouch and faceplate

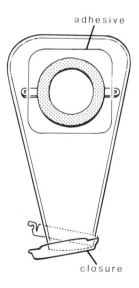

adhesive

closure

FIG. 18. Standard ileostomy appliance.

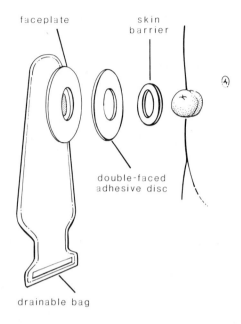

faceplate   skin barrier

double-faced adhesive disc

drainable bag

FIG. 19. Reusable ileostomy appliance.

can be cleaned and reused; the adhesive gasket and skin barrier are replaced at each change. It is advisable to have two sets of reusable equipment and to rotate usage. Such equipment can last indefinitely with proper care.

The advantages of reusable equipment are (a) decreased cost—the main portion of the system is reused; (b) custom fit—the equipment can accommodate any uneven areas that may cause disposable systems to lift away from the skin; and (c) increased wearing time—the faceplate does not melt away after 4 to 5 days as the skin barrier will with the disposable equipment.

COLOSTOMY

The colon is approximately 5 to 6 feet in length and is divided into six sections: the cecum, ascending colon, transverse colon, descending colon, sigmoid colon, and rectum (see Fig. 20). A colostomy is a surgically created opening into the colon in one side of the five sections above the cecum. The location of the colostomy opening, or stoma, depends on the underlying reason for surgery.

Several different types of colostomies can be created. A single-opening or end colostomy is created by bringing the colon out through an opening in the skin. The colon is either sewn flush to the skin or inverted (folded over on itself) and attached to the skin. A double-barreled colostomy has two openings, one that discharges stool (the active stoma) and one that leads to the resting or dysfunctional colon (the mucus fistula). The loop colostomy is a loop of bowel that is brought out through an opening on the skin. The loop of colon is held in place with a rod or bridge underneath it until it heals onto the skin (usually 5–10 days) (Fig. 21).

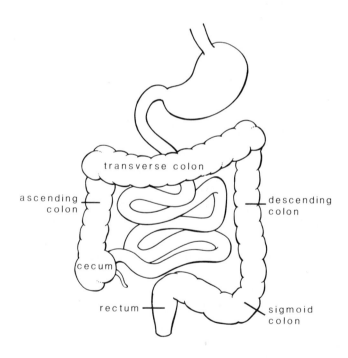

FIG. 20. Anatomy of the colon.

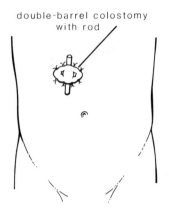

double-barrel colostomy
with rod

FIG. 21. Double-barrel colostomy.

Since water is reabsorbed from the stool along the length of the colon, the quality of the colostomy output depends on the length of the intact large bowel. For instance, a colostomy on the right side of the colon (ascending colon) discharges liquid contents at frequent intervals not unlike an ileostomy, whereas stool from a sigmoid colostomy (left-sided) may be discharged less frequently as formed material because the greater length of colon yet remaining allows the reabsorption of salt and water.

Placement of the colostomy stoma on the abdomen is important (see placement of ileostomy). The optimum location allows the person flexibility in movement and activities. Preoperatively, the stoma site is selected by the surgeon and the enterostomal nurse therapist.

The colostomy stoma varies in size depending on the type created and the location in the colon. It will also have a red, moist appearance similar to the lining inside the mouth. Like the ileostomy, the colostomy imparts no pain when touched, and there is no sensation when stool passes out. Thus, an appliance or pouch is usually worn over the colostomy to collect the stool. In some patients with left-sided colostomies the stool output may be "trained" to occur daily (sometimes after breakfast or a simple irrigation), so that only a small patch or single dressing is needed to cover the stoma.

Care of Colostomy

Postoperatively, the colostomy is cared for in the same manner as the ileostomy (see care of ileostomy). A skin barrier is worn to protect the skin against the stool, and a drainable pouch is used. After healing takes place (usually 4–6 weeks), left-sided colostomies may have stool passing once a day or less. In this case, the stool is formed and not harmful to the skin, and the skin barrier may not be necessary.

Long-term management of ascending and transverse colostomies generally requires the use of appropriate skin barriers and drainable disposable pouches. Reusable equipment, contrary to the situation with ileostomies, is not advisable because of the presence of bacteria in the colon.

Irrigation is an option available to some people with a left-sided colostomy. Water is put into the colon through an irrigation set (similar to an enema kit), which cleanses the colon of stool. This is done at the same time every day in order to "train" the colon only to eliminate stool when water is placed in it. The goal of irrigation is to have no stool pass out between daily irrigations. The person who is successful with irrigation wears a pad or small pouch over the stoma between irrigations. Colostomy irrigation is considered an option in the management of colostomies and is by no means necessary to maintain its function.

DIET

In response to the operation, the stoma can be expected to be swollen for some time. This swelling (edema) can last 6 to 8 weeks after surgery. The edema causes the stomal opening to be temporarily smaller than its eventual size, and certain foods can block the stoma as they pass out. As a result, some foods must be avoided for the first 6 to 8 weeks or until the stoma has "matured." The foods to be avoided contain undigestable vegetable fiber, which can clump or "ball-up," and include nuts, corn, popcorn, chinese vegetables, mushrooms, and celery. After the edema has subsided, these foods are gradually introduced one at a time but should always be well chewed. If discomfort (cramps, distention) or a diminished ostomy output is noted, they should be avoided.

In general, there are few dietary restrictions for the person with an ileostomy or colostomy. In the beginning, foods that have not been eaten for some time should be tried one at a time and in small amounts. If no problems are noted, these can be added to the diet. Since the colon is responsible for absorbing fluid from the ingested food, when all or a portion of the colon has been removed, additional fluids may be necessary to compensate and allow adequate hydration. Extra fluids will be administered initially (for a short time) after surgery until the body begins to adjust to the loss of the colon. Then the thirst mechanism will take over to let the person know when additional fluid is needed.

ACTIVITY

A stoma will not limit a person from participation in almost any activity he or she may choose. Certain contact sports may be restricted because of the possibility of a direct blow to the stoma or slippage of the pouch. As long as the appliance is well sealed against the skin, most activities should not dislodge the seal. Running, tennis, and golf, as well as other sports, can be enjoyed with no problems.

Swimming, bathing, and showering should present no worry about the appliance coming off. Many of the pouches have waterproof adhesive tape. For those that do not, waterproof tape can be placed around the edge of the pouch adhesive to seal out the water. Showering or bathing may be done with the appliance off if desired. The peristomal area can be thoroughly cleansed, and there will be no problems with the soap or water touching or entering the stoma.

To support the ostomy appliance under a swimsuit, a light stretch panty for women or jockey-styled underwear for men can be worn. The undergarment aids in flattening the pouch against the body.

The concept of undergarments flattening the appliance under a swimsuit also may be employed when wearing clothes. Loose or baggy clothes allow the pouch to puff out, causing a noticeable bulge. Undergarments should be form fitted, and the appliance worn beneath the underwear. Frequently, because of the length of the pouch, it is folded, and the clamp placed at the fold of the thigh. The underwear is then brought up over the pouch, holding it in place. The stool will drain into the pouch but will be distributed throughout instead of filling up the bottom. Snug clothes will not prevent the stoma from draining. Belts should not ride directly on the stoma, since the friction may irritate the stoma and loosen the appliance. An ostomy should not limit clothing options; there will be few if any restrictions on the style of clothes.

ADJUSTMENTS

Physically, living with a stoma is not difficult. It necessitates wearing an appliance and learning how to work with the necessary equipment. The mechanics are easily learned and mastered so that even most children can attend to their own appliances. Some mental adjustment is needed in dealing with a change in the way the body functions. It takes time and the support of friends or family to help an individual adjust to the concept of a stoma and the fear of social rejection.

Adjustment appears to take place in stages. Initially, much of the postoperative time and energy is spent working with the stoma and equipment. After actually touching the stoma and handling the equipment, the body change begins to be personalized: it becomes part of one's self. Once a person learns how to change and empty the appliance, confidence builds, and adjustment progresses.

The next stage occurs when the significant other, the wife, husband, child, or friend, is told and/or shown the stoma. Their reaction, interest, and acceptance will help in the personal adjustment.

The third stage or phase of adjustment is social contact—going to school, work, or out shopping. It is now that the person tests whether the pouch will really stay on when he or she gets out of the car or climbs up the steps. It is now that it is tested whether others really know, or if any type of clothing can be worn.

All of these stages contribute to a feeling of well-being, but as with any adjustments, it takes patience, time, and understanding. What is most important is that the person feels in control—the rest will follow.

SEX

Sexuality is a combination of feelings that one expresses in various ways. The way a person perceives oneself contributes to his or her sexual being. After ostomy surgery, much energy is used in the healing process and in learning how to deal physically with the stoma and necessary equipment. In contrast, the physical illness will usually have been improved, and the accompanying strain on the patient's physical and mental energy should be lifted. Gradually, a sense of well-being is reestablished, and the ostomate begins to feel comfortable with the stoma and equipment. This is the time when one may question how the stoma will affect his or her sexual functioning.

The surgeon usually approves of sexual activity once the abdominal and/or perineal wound is healed. This usually corresponds to a 4 to 6 week period after surgery, when the patient is otherwise recovering and rarely feeling the "urge" for sex. Again, patience is essential for both the ostomate and partner in realizing this essential recuperative interval and that the initial lack of interest on the patient's part is normal. Needless to say, after any surgery (or after having a baby for that matter), the initial encounter needs to be extraordinarily gentle as the couple gains confidence in the way the body will function and to avoid any postoperative stiffness or discomfort near the incision.

Unless the stoma is regulated by irrigation, the appliance remains on during sex. It is advisable to empty the appliance prior to any activity, decreasing the risk of the pouch detaching from the skin. Aside from emptying the pouch prior to sex, no special arrangements need to be taken. Some people prefer to tape the pouch against the body to avoid its moving around or to use a cloth cover over the appliance. These are personal habits depending on each individual.

Confidence is achieved during lovemaking if the ostomate knows that his or her appliance is leakproof and odor-free. This confidence must be shared with the sexual partner by explaining to him or her that close physical contact (i.e., hugging, body pressure against the abdomen) will not hurt the stoma or cause the appliance to detach from the skin. Acceptance by the sexual partner increases the osto-mate's confidence, and things should proceed smoothly.

Women with a stoma can have safe and healthy pregnancies and deliveries. Some doctors may advise a 1- to 2-year period of adjust-ment after surgery before conception. The stoma will not interfere with a normal delivery. As the abdomen enlarges with the preg-nancy, adjustments may need to be made in the appliance, but these are generally minor. Of course, women should consult their per-sonal physicians/surgeons regarding these recommendations for an individual case.

RESOURCES

There are resources available for the person anticipating or having had ostomy surgery. The United Ostomy Association is a nation-wide group, the purpose of which is to offer support and information to anyone who is interested. There are local chapters in nearly every community that have monthly educational meetings and a visitor's group. The visitor's group is made up of trained ostomy visitors who visit patients in the hospital anticipating or recovering from surgery. They can offer support just by their normal physical appearance, by walking into a person's room looking healthy, wear-ing clothes, and understanding what the patient is going through emotionally and physically.

The United Ostomy Association publishes several pamphlets, booklets, and a quarterly magazine on ostomy-related subjects. The magazine, *The Ostomy Quarterly*, carries information on the newest ostomy equipment as well as articles of interest to all ostomates (see Appendix for information on the Ostomy Association).

Another important resource is the enterostomal nurse therapist. Enterostomal nurse therapists are professional nurses who have postgraduate education in the ostomy field. They work with osto-mates and medical professionals in all phases of ostomy care and rehabilitation. The enterostomal nurse specialist can provide pre-operative consultation (including the choice stoma site), postopera-tive instruction on how to choose and use the correct equipment, on fitting, and on skin care essentials, and continuous education through the stoma or surgery clinic, after the patient has been discharged from the hospital. The International Association for Enterostomal Therapy can be contacted for referrals and additional information (see Appendix).

APPENDIX

Organizations

United Ostomy Association, Inc.
2001 W. Beverly Boulevard
Los Angeles, CA 90057
(213) 413-5510

Some publications available:

1. The Ostomy Quarterly
2. Ileostomies: A Guide
3. Colostomies: A Guide
4. Urinary Ostomies: A Guidebook for Patients
5. Sex, Courtship and the Single Ostomate
6. Sex and the Male Ostomate
7. Sex and the Female Ostomate
8. Pregnancy and the Woman with an Ostomy

International Association for Enterstomal Therapy
1 Newport Place
Suite 970
Newport Beach, CA 92660
(714) 476-0268

Publications

1. *The Ostomy Book*. Barbara D. Mullen and Kerry Anne McGinn. Bull Publishing Co., 1980, Palo Alto, CA.
2. *These Special Children: The Ostomy Book for Parents of Children with Colostomies, Ileostomies, and Urostomies*. Katherine F. Jeter, EdD, E.T. Bull Publishing Co., 1982, Palo Alto, CA.

Manufacturers of Ostomy Equipment

Hollister Incorporated
2000 Hollister Drive
Libertyville, IL 60048

Convatec
E. R. Squibb
P.O. Box 4000
Princeton, N.J. 08540

United
Hawmedica, Inc.
11775 Starkey Rd.
Largo, FL 33543

John F. Greer Company
530 E. 12th Street
Oakland, CA 94606

Nu Hope Laboratories, Inc.
P. O. Box 39348
Los Angeles, CA 90039

Bard Home Health Division
C. R. Bard, Inc.
Berkeley Heights, N.J. 07922

Marlen Manufacturing & Development Co.
5150 Richmond Road
Bedford, OH 44146

CHAPTER 14

Future Directions

Until the exact cause(s) and the eventual cure for the inflammatory bowel diseases have been determined, research will continue along various lines. A major roadblock in research related to inflammatory bowel disease has been the absence of a true animal model. Inflammatory disease of the bowel similar to that in humans has yet to be produced in animals. This has left a major gap in the search for potential infectious agents, toxins, and the testing of new drugs prior to trials with humans. Unlike some illnesses that can be studied in animals, inflammatory bowel disease, to this date, appears to be unique to man. Current studies attempting to transmit inflammatory bowel disease from humans to animals include feeding a new bacterium, mycobacteria, to pygmy goats and investigating the cause of colitis in the cotton-top marmoset.

A major research interest continues to be an infectious agent or agents. Many bacterial infections of the gastrointestinal tract cannot be differentiated from inflammatory bowel disease clinically over a short period of time because of identical or similar changes in the tissues. Many instances of what turn out to be idiopathic inflammatory bowel disease also appear to be initiated by intestinal infections. However, no documented infection is known to persist with the identical chronic course of either ulcerative colitis or Crohn's disease. It is the continuation of symptoms in the absence of known disease-producing infections that distinguishes inflammatory bowel disease. Therefore, studies with viruses, bacteria of various types, and parasitic agents have proved negative. On the other hand, there are so many different bacterial species that continued efforts in this direction are justified.

A considerable amount of time and money has been concentrated on the search for an immunologic cause of inflammatory bowel disease. The gut immune system is so intricately related to protection against invasion by infectious agents and gut toxins that alterations in the intestinal immune system would be a logical source of the difficulty. Abnormalities have been identified in the immune system in patients, but only after inflammatory bowel disease has been established. Therefore, no immunologic dysfunction has been recognized *prior* to the onset of inflammatory bowel disease, but studies of this type have yet to be undertaken. Continued research is necessary to further understand the complex development and the multiple interrelationships of the gut immune system, food allergy, other allergic phenomena, the handling of toxins, and the overall immune defenses of the host. The continuity with the entire immune system is exemplified by the potential extraintestinal symptoms such as skin rashes, arthritis, and eye problems, which may complicate the course of inflammatory bowel disease.

Additional work is also needed in the area of the inflammatory response in general. As we begin to understand the complex biochemical nature of inflammation within other tissues, newer methods of controlling these reactions in the gut should become apparent.

Research related to genetics and the family occurrence of inflammatory bowel disease will continue to be oriented to the question of whether or not inflammatory bowel disease is caused by environmental factors or whether the illness is a biologic process completely determined on a genetic basic. Extended observations of family members and relatives who develop inflammatory bowel disease may be able to discriminate a mode of inheritance such that prevention, early intervention, or genetic counseling may eventually be available. Additional work in the area of molecular biology (studying the individual genetic material that forms the foundation of all the cellular reactions within the body) will be directed at identifying the genes responsible for the immune response and may allow more precise diagnoses and genetic manipulation over the course of an illness.

Advances in the field of nutrition also are important for the further understanding of inflammatory bowel disease. Studies of dietary factors both before and after the onset of inflammatory bowel disease may identify potential initiating or aggravating factors that may be controlled or utilized to prevent the occurrence of inflammatory bowel disease. As yet, no specific food has definitely been implicated in patients who eventually develop inflammatory bowel disease, nor are any dietary factors known to cause an inflammatory response in man. Further work is necessary to clarify this complex area of investigation.

Progress also continues to be made related to new therapies of inflammatory bowel disease. Newer antibiotics continue to be developed that may eventually help towards the identification of potential infectious agents. Likewise, the increased understanding of why current therapies are (or are not) effective in inflammatory bowel disease continues to improve. As 5-ASA has been recognized as the effective ingredient in sulfasalazine, newer methods of delivering this drug to the involved tissues are evolving. New drugs affecting the inflammatory response are under investigation. Newer steroid agents that will act with a potent antiinflammatory action but without the well-known side effects should soon be available. Medications that will alter the immune response are also being actively studied. Our understanding of nutrition in inflammatory bowel disease also has received considerable attention. Hyperalimentation and bowel rest can be important adjuncts in the treatment, yet the mechanism by which they are effective is still under study. Continued efforts in regard to the benefits of resting the bowel and methods to assess the effects of bowel rest on the gut immune system are needed in order to better understand the relationships of the intestinal tract with its environment.

In order to continue work in the field of inflammatory bowel disease, two important ingredients are necessary. The first is dissemination of knowledge about the problem of inflammatory bowel disease. If these illnesses are kept in the "closet," little public information will be directed to these problems, and interest will be limited to those families with an affected individual. Enhanced efforts to publicize inflammatory bowel disease, the difficulties it presents, and the expense (emotional and physical as well as financial) related to the treatment are essential. Second, money is required to support scientific investigations. The Federal Government currently is providing only limited funds for research on IBD. Private foundations and other sources of public support need to be developed to provide sufficient support for this very important objective.

At the present time, there are several organizations that directly sponsor research in inflammatory bowel disease. The foremost is the National Foundation for Ileitis and Colitis. This organization functions at both national and local levels to provide financial support for research. It also provides educational material for patients and their families. Other local agencies such as the Gastrointestinal Research Foundation of Chicago sponsor research related to inflammatory bowel disease at the University of Chicago. Several pharmaceutical companies also are directly involved in supporting the evaluation of possible therapeutic agents.

Despite the considerable activity by these and other organizations, the total effort remains limited. We, physicians and patients, fervently await the day when the cause and the cure of IBD will be at hand and, like so many other now-eliminated diseases, inflammatory bowel disease, too, will become of only historical interest. Until this time, medical professionals and the public will continue their cooperative efforts to eliminate and control these challenging disorders.

Glossary

Abscess: A pocket of pus or localized collection of inflammatory tissue.

Adhesion: Fibrous scar tissue that interconnects (adheres to) two structures (e.g., two loops of intestines or intestine to the abdominal wall).

Amino acids: The single units that, when linked together, produce proteins.

Amylase: An enzyme produced by the pancreas and salivary glands that digests complex sugars and starches.

Anabolic: The metabolic process through which muscle mass and protein are increased; the opposite of catabolic.

Anastomosis: A surgical connection.

Ankylosing spondylitis: A form of arthritis involving the spine that is seen occasionally in patients with IBD and eventually leads to a stiffening, or straightening, of the back.

Antibody: Substances produced by immune cells that recognize foreign material (antigens) and bind to them so that they may be eliminated or destroyed by other immune cells.

Anticholinergic: Drugs that relax the smooth muscle of the intestine.

Antigen: Any material that, in a sensitive person, causes the body tissues to react to destroy or eliminate the substance.

Anus (anal sphincter): The last segment of the digestive tract at the junction of the rectum in the skin composed of a combination of voluntary and involuntary circular muscle fibers that maintain the closure of the rectum.

Aphthous: A minute, circular ulcer overlying a lymphoid follicle as in aphthoid ulcer. The earliest visible feature of Crohn's disease that occurs in the mouth or intestine.

Autoimmune reaction: An inflammatory reaction against one's own body tissues. The reaction can be very specific such as against a single protein or DNA.

Barium enema: An X-ray examination of the colon, also referred to as a lower GI.

Catheter: A tube or hollow pipe that is entered into a body organ such as into the bladder (Foley catheter) or into a vein (i.v. catheter).

Cecum: The first portion of the large intestine.

Cellulose: A common form of plant fiber that makes up the majority of plant cell walls and is composed of glucose units linked by a special chemical bond that human beings are unable to digest.

Chymotrypsin: One of the variety of digestive enzymes that breaks down protein into smaller segments.

Clubbing: Refers to changes in the fingernails or toenails with an elevation or rounding up of the nail plate.

Coenzyme: A chemical that is necessary for an enzyme to be effective. Usually these are minerals (trace elements) that are required by the body in minute amounts, but without which the biochemical systems of the individual cells will not function.

Colectomy: The removal of a portion (or all) of the colon.

Colonoscope: A long, flexible instrument used to examine the entire colon and terminal ileum.

Colostomy: A surgically created opening of the colon onto the skin.

Corticosteroid: Any of a variety of medications derived from the hormone cortisone (hydrocortisone, prednisone, methylprednisone, etc.).

Cushing's disease: The condition of having excess cortisone in the body that is manifest as a rounded ''moon face'', a redistribution of fat to the torso and abdomen, a thinning of the skin with occasional purple streaks (striae), a thinning of the bones, increased blood pressure, etc.

Duodenum: The first portion of the small intestine after the stomach into which the bile and pancreatic secretions enter.

Dysplasia: Refers to tissue in which the individual cells have become atypical or precancerous.

Edema: A collection of tissue fluids that produces swelling either in the skin or any body organ.

Endoscopic: Refers to an examination through an endoscope, such as a gastroscope or colonoscope.

Enteral: Refers to foods or medicine administered through the mouth or intestinal tract.

Enteroclysis: A special method of performing X-rays of the small intestine in which the barium is administered through a tube rather than swallowed directly.

Enterostomal therapist: A nurse who specializes in the care of ostomy patients.

Enzyme: A protein chemical that accelerates reactions to break down other chemicals.

Erythema nodosum: Painful, dusky-blue nodules occasionally associated with IBD, occurring most commonly over the shins.

Esophagus: The segment of the digestive tract between the mouth and stomach.

Extraintestinal: Pertains to symptoms or abnormalities not directly related to the GI tract.

Fissure: A crack, crevice or longitudinal ulcer.

Fistula: An abnormal tract connecting two structures.

Follicle: A cluster or grouping of cells; usually lymphocytes as a lymphoid follicle.

Friability: Pertains to tissue that breaks apart or bleeds after minor manipulation.

Gastroesophageal junction: The anatomic valve between the esophagus and stomach.

Glucose: A simple sugar which provides the building block for many more complex sugars and carbohydrates.

Granuloma: A specific pathologic feature of Crohn's disease where "giant cells" are seen in the tissues.

Granulomatis colitis: A synonym for Crohn's disease of the colon as compared with ulcerative colitis.

Growth hormone: A chemical secreted by the pituitary gland which stimulates the growth of bones and tissues.

Hyperalimentation: The adminstration of a large amount of calories and nutritional substances, whether through a vein or intestinal tube.

Idiopathic: A disease of unknown cause.

Ileocolitis: Crohn's disease involving both the small and large intestines.

Ileostomy: A surgically created opening of the ileum onto the skin.

Ileum: The second half of the small intestine that enters into the colon as the terminal ileum.

Iritis: Inflammation of the iris of the eye producing a painful, pink-eye.

Jejunoileitis: Usually applies to Crohn's disease limited to the small intestine involving both the jejunum and ileum.

Jejunum: The first half of the small intestine.

Lactase: The enzyme that breaks apart the milk-sugar lactose into its two components, glucose and galactose. This enzyme sits on the cells lining the small intestine.

Lactose: Milk-sugar; a disaccharide (double-sugar) composed of glucose and galactose.

Large intestine: The large bowel or colon, which is composed of the appendix, cecum, ascending colon, transverse colon, descending colon, sigmoid colon, and rectum.

Lipase: A digestive enzyme produced by the pancreas that breaks down fat globules into smaller subunits (fatty acids).

Lumen: The inside of a tubular organ.

Lymphocytes: A variety of white blood cells that carries immunologic activity.

Macrophage: A white blood cell that acts as a scavenger in "cleaning up" harmful substances in tissue.

Mast cell: A white blood cell that releases histamine in allergic reactions to produce hives or local tissue injury.

Metastasis: Spread beyond the original location, usually referring to the spread of a tumor to distant sites.

Mucosa: The innermost lining of the digestive tract.

Mucus: The clear secretion of the digestive tract that acts as a normal lubricant of the intestines.

Nidus: The initial point of origin of a process (e.g., the nidus of an infection).

Nodule: A swelling or lump.

Osteomalacia: Bone disease due to an inadequate supply of vitamin D. Insufficient amounts of calcium are incorporated into the bone material leaving soft and weakened bones.

Ostomy: Synonym for stoma, a surgically created opening of the intestine usually to the skin.

Oxalate: A chemical found in many fruits and leafy vegetables that is absorbed in unusually large amounts in patients who have malabsorption of fat. After absorption into the bloodstream from the colon, the oxalate can be eliminated in the urinary system where it frequently causes kidney and bladder stones.

Pancolitis: Inflammation involving the entire colon from the rectum to the cecum.

Pancreas: An abdominal gland that produces a variety of hormones (insulin and glucagon) as well as digestive enzymes, which are secreted into the duodenum and there mix with the liquid contents leaving the stomach.

Parenteral: Refers to the administration of medicines or foods by any method except through the mouth or intestine (e.g., an intramuscular injection or through an intravenous route).

Paresthesia: A tingling or funny sensation usually in the fingers, hands, toes, or feet.

Pepsin: One of several digestive enzymes that breaks down protein chains into smaller segments.

Perforation: Pertaining to a tear, leak, or rupture usually of an inflamed portion of the intestine or appendix.

Perianal: Located around the anus.

Pericholangitis: A minor liver abnormality seen frequently in inflammatory bowel disease, usually manifest as a slight elevation of liver blood tests (usually alkaline phosphatase).

Perineal: The area of the lower abdomen between the genitals and anus.

Peristalsis: The muscular activity of the digestive tract that propels food down the length of the tube.

Peritoneal cavity: The membrane that encloses the abdominal organs beneath the layers of the abdominal wall.

Plasma cells: A form of white blood cells that produce antibodies.

Polymorphonuclear leukocytes: A form of white blood cells that are active in protecting the body from harmful infectious agents (pus cells).

Polyp: A growth on the lining of the intestine that may be either be benign or malignant (cancerous).

Pouchitis: Inflammation within a surgically created intestinal pouch (e.g., in a Koch's pouch or ileal reservoir).

Proctitis: Inflammation of the rectum.

Proctocolectomy: The removal of the entire colon and rectum.

Proctoscope: A straight, metal tube with a light on one end used to examine the rectum.

Pylorus: The sphincter between the stomach and duodenum.

Pyoderma gangrenosum: A severe skin lesion occasionally seen in patients with inflammatory bowel disease that occurs as an ulcerating sore most commonly on the legs.

Rectum: The final segment of the large intestine (colon).

Regional enteritis: A synonym for Crohn's disease of the intestine.

Sacroiliitis: A form of arthritis of the spine that occasionally is seen in patients with inflammatory bowel disease and leads to symptoms of low back pain.

Sclerosing cholangitis: A severe form of liver disease that rarely accompanies ulcerative colitis, involving a blockage of the bile ducts in the liver thus leading to more severe liver disease (cirrhosis).

Serosal: The outermost layer of the intestines and digestive organs.

Sigmoidoscope: A flexible instrument used to examine the lower third of the colon and rectum.

Smooth muscle: A specialized form of muscle that surrounds the digestive organs (esophagus, stomach, and intestines).

Somatomedin: A chemical messenger that interacts with growth hormone to stimulate growth.

Sphincter: Muscular tissue arranged in a circular array to clamp down or hold a tubular structure closed.

Splenic flexure: The bend in the colon at the junction of the transverse and descending colons located just beneath the spleen.

Stoma: A surgically created opening of intestine to the skin. Examples are a colostomy, when the colon is brought out to the skin or an ileostomy, when the ileum is brought out to the skin.

Stomach: The segment of the digestive tract between the esophagus and duodenum that acts as a reservoir into which acid and digestive enzymes are secreted to break down large chunks of food.

Stricture: A narrowing, usually produced by active inflammation or scar tissue.

Submucosa: The layer of the digestive tract beneath the mucosa that contains supporting and structural elements of the bowel.

Tenesmus: A severe crampy sensation in the lower abdomen associated with the urge to defecate.

Terminal ileitis: A synonym for Crohn's disease of the ileum or regional enteritis.

Terminal ileum: The last segment of the small intestine, which enters into the cecum at the ileocecal valve. This segment is important for the absorption of vitamin B-12, fat soluble vitamins, and bile salts.

Toxic megacolon: A severe condition occurring in either Crohn's disease or ulcerative colitis in which the colon rapidly dilates, the walls become very thin, and there is a susceptability to perforation or rupture.

Ulceration: The formation of an ulcer, a wound with the loss of surface tissues in any part of the body.

Ulcerative proctitis: A variant of ulcerative colitis in which the inflammation does not extend beyond the rectum.

Uric acid: A chemical end product of protein metabolism that can crystallize in the joints (causing gout) or urinary tract (producing kidney stones).

Urostomy: A surgically created diversion of the urinary system onto the skin.

Uveitis: Inflammation of the inner portions of the eye similar to iritis, producing a red, sore eye with occasional blurred vision.

Villus (pl. villi): The tiny folds of the small intestine that greatly increase the absorptive surface area of the small bowel.

Subject Index